What people are saying about

Awakening the Lotus of Peace

Yoga has become very popular around the world, but many people practise yoga simply as an exercise to keep fit. Jenny Light's book is a guide to practise yoga to find peace and harmony within and in the world. *Awakening the Lotus of Peace* helps the reader to underst⌐⌐ ɔiritual and practical yoga. I hope everᵧ ˙ad this book and be inspired to r er peace and outer peace.

Satish Kuma ⌐esurgence & Ecologist Magazine

This latest offering from Jenny Light is a balm for the soul. An exquisite mix of practical advice on the how-tos of meditation, coupled with spiritual wisdom on the true purpose of life: finding lasting happiness and peace with God. Gleaned from attunement and communion with her Guru Paramahansa Yogananda; this book is a treasure trove for devotees around the world and those seeking deeper meaning to life. In a world of constant flux, Jenny offers an antidote: peace. Within its pages you will discover 15 separate meditations on aspects of peace, yoga breathing techniques, exercises in introspection and much more.

Anita Neilson, author of *Soul Murmurs: Seasonal words of spiritual wisdom to enlighten the soul* (O-Books 2019)

If you dream of a happy, successful life, where the worries of the world cannot ruffle your feathers, then this book is for you. Jenny Light shares her yogic wisdom through easy to follow breathing and meditation practices, and her own deeply touching life experiences.

Whether you're well-practised, or completely new to meditation, Jenny's honest and humane storytelling delivers a profound knowledge of peace, accessible to everyone. As I read this book, I felt instantly calmer and more able to deal with life's trials and uncertainties. It offers practical solutions to stop the internal chatter in your head and disastrous drive of the ego.

This work is a balm for all who need peace in troubled times, and a much needed cleansing workout for your lungs, sinuses and soul.

Allison Galbraith, Author of *Dancing with Trees: Eco Tales from the British Isles*. The History Press, 2017 & Lanarkshire Folktales, 2021

Right from the first page, as I began to read, I sensed a feeling of calm and gentleness. The very words used and the ebb and flow of the writing led to me begin in a more relaxed state, even as I read those first few pages.

I found the thoughts on ego and how to overcome it and live more in a soul-based state incredibly interesting and I could see on reflection how I could have handled things in my own past differently to achieve a more peaceful outcome. It has already started to change my perspective in a very short time.

Awakening the Lotus of Peace is the perfect mix of expression, experience and detailed exercises to help you get to grips with your own path to soul and peace. Jenny has a wonderful way with words and has crafted something beautiful and befitting of the topic.

Laura Bland, Author and Speaker, Laura B Empowered Words

Throughout this book, Jenny's devotion to and gratitude to her guru and her practice of meditation shine through. Sincerely felt words tell us of the benefits of meditation and remind us of our deep need and yearning for the spiritual peace that it bestows.

Awakening the Lotus of Peace is a treasure trove of many things; advice on the importance of true peace in our lives; prayers and mantras, meditations and exercises to help us reach that blissful state. All draw on a blend of ancient practices and Jenny's own experience as both practitioner and teacher. Moving and inspiring in equal measures.

Jane Hill, modern mystic, author of *Six Enchantments* (Amethyst Living 2020)

This most recent book from Jenny was inspired by a poem on 'Peace' by her guru Paramahansa Yogananda. It is a composite of divine channelling from him together with wisdom gained by Jenny over her many years of spiritual practice and her experience in yoga, psychology and philosophy. It contains numerous practical techniques, visualisation, affirmation, mantras, prayers, yoga breathing exercises and meditations to assist the reader to master meditation and to help achieve inner peace with the ultimate goal of divine communion with source. This goal is not easily achieved but requires patience, persistence and perseverance. In Jenny's words we should 'keep on keeping on' until we achieve our desired goal.
James McPherson, Meditation Student

Whether you are a seasoned Yogi or Meditator or new to meditation, you will enjoy this book. Even just reading through this book without following any of the meditations I felt an instant feeling of calmness and peace.

As you journey through this book you will be taught techniques to calm the monkey mind, move aside ego and focus on your goal: Peace. You will be taught how to prepare the body prior to meditation: Relax the body and the mind will follow. With 15 separate meditations, there really is something for everyone, regardless of your experience. As you move through the meditations the author will gently guide you through each step, instructing you on breathing techniques, focus and visualisations.

This book has kick-started my daily meditations (again!), although this time, I have to say, something has changed. I genuinely feel more peaceful, more tolerant and more focused on finding my true-self and purpose.

Thank you Jenny for bringing together all your experience and taking the time to write this book. It is a book that I will certainly return to and the contents of which I will certainly share within my Yoga & Qi Gong classes.

Donna McKeown, Yoga and Qi Gong teacher

In this book Jenny helps describe how control of the breath, and gaining mental focus through detaching the mind and practising meditation, leads to a deep calm stillness and peace. Her great insights, practical hints and methods for meditation make achieving the calm state of mind accessible to anyone. The exercises are described in a comprehensive way to encourage control of the body and the breath. Jenny describes the theory and reasons behind this process in a clear and comprehensive way, and provides many tools and methods for both beginners and experienced meditators to try. Staying present, watching the breath is available to anyone and I thoroughly recommend this book, which consolidates all I have learned whilst practising meditation with Jenny over the past four years.

Caroline Mitchell, Yoga Teacher

If you are fortunate enough to get your hands on this book, you may well be on your way to changing your life forever. My mentor and the author of this book, Jenny Light, has guided me through some very toxic and chaotic situations in my life. Before I met Jenny, I am not proud to say, I was a very dissatisfied, unhappy, anxious and stressed-out selfish person, who really didn't care much for anyone or anything other than myself. I drank too much, smoked like a lum, ate too much rubbish and worked myself into a frenzy. I really was a crazy 40-something woman trying to keep up in this marathon of life and drowning my sorrow at the weekend, to wake up after a 3-day hangover and look forward to the following weekend. Barely an existence.

If you think you are past your sell-by date to change your life, if you are at the end of your tether or if you just need some meaning in your life then this book and Jenny's teachings are perfect for you.

Forget all the self-help or counselling books, I have read most of them. If you seriously want to find true happiness, inner peace and live a fulfilled life, then this book is the key.

Thank you for showing me this path, Jenny, all your continued support and teaching me this beautiful way of life.
Linsey McLean, Meditation Student

As a newbie to Yoga Meditation I found this book truly fulfilling and inspirational, not only on a spiritual level, however, as it also brought an amazing blissful Peace into my personal life which is much needed during the 'craziness' of current times.

Concentrating on the beautifully illustrated mandalas in the book provides the essential pre-requisite of single-pointed focus to fully experience these peace-infused Yoga meditations which can be achieved by everyone. Yoga practice is a commitment which must be continuously followed, the benefits and changes that can be made to your life are mind-blowing!
Marlene McPherson, Meditation Student

Awakening the Lotus of Peace

Yoga Meditation for Inner Peace

Awakening the Lotus of Peace

Yoga Meditation for Inner Peace

Jenny Light

Illustrations by Lesley Brown

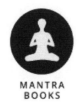

MANTRA
BOOKS

Winchester, UK
Washington, USA

JOHN HUNT PUBLISHING

First published by Mantra Books, 2022
Mantra Books is an imprint of John Hunt Publishing Ltd., No. 3 East Street, Alresford
Hampshire SO24 9EE, UK
office@jhpbooks.com
www.johnhuntpublishing.com
www.mantra-books.net

For distributor details and how to order please visit the 'Ordering' section on our website.

Text copyright: Jenny Light 2020

ISBN: 978 1 78904 887 2
978 1 78904 888 9 (ebook)
Library of Congress Control Number: 2021932916

A CIP catalogue record for this book is available from the British Library.

Design: Stuart Davies

UK: Printed and bound by CPI Group (UK) Ltd, Croydon, CR0 4YY
Printed in North America by CPI GPS partners

We operate a distinctive and ethical publishing philosophy in
all areas of our business, from our global network of authors to
production and worldwide distribution.

Contents

Preface

One late November day in 2018, I was in rapture, meditating on the poem 'Peace' by Paramahansa Yogananda, from his book *Metaphysical Meditations*, when out of the blue I heard the voice of my divine guru speaking to me in the quiet of meditation. The buzz of my mind had become still and I could hear his clear, insistent voice encouraging me to write this book. He imparted to me his wish that I reach as many souls as possible with the vibration of peace. He promised to bring his aid to each of you who connects with him and meditates on his poetic Peace poem. He showed me that each phrase is imbued with seed wisdom which he wanted me to help make accessible, broken down into fifteen separate meditations for the first time.

Filled with the light of illumination from the guru, this task seemed easy but later doubts assailed me. Pouring out my heart to God, I said: *Why do you wish me to write this book on Peace? I who have so little of this quality and who is often beset with restlessness? I know that you are Peace itself but that peace is often hidden from me and I lose you in the mental and physical clamour. Please guide me, Lord. I need your peace, your over-shadowing protection and your presence. No more do I wish a garment of jangling restlessness. Instead, Lord, bring your balm of peace to soothe my nerves, my mind, my cares. I lay a sweet-perfumed offering of my soul-flower to fragrance Thy Halls of Peace. Let my soul be found in grace to walk the halls of Thy mansion in Peace.*

And a Peace came upon me and I understood at last what Peace is. Words are totally inadequate to describe the deep rest that comes when the restlessness within is at last still. It is like drinking the sweetest most refreshing water after walking in a parched wilderness or finally having blessed sleep after weeks of stressful unrest.

Much of the material for this book has been channelled

1

through me during my meditation classes to my students. In my own humble words, I have tried to impart that living vibration of Peace within this book as accessible through easy yoga breathing techniques and scripted meditations. This book is offered in deepest gratitude to God, my revered guru, Paramahansa Yogananda, and the faithful support of my students.

Introduction

Peace is a quality which is universal in its appeal. When we tire of the allure and strife of the material world, young or old, the desire is then for peace, as peace is the true state of the soul. Quietly calling in the depth of our being we may be aware that we have lost something very dear and precious. In a quiet inner knowing, there is the recognition that living life in a constant hurry and driving ourselves hard to achieve earthly goals is somehow empty. No matter how much we do, or push or achieve, there just never seems to be an end to it. And all the while, quietly in our heart of hearts, there is the longing for inner peace. All that earthly striving avails nothing. Each summit of achievement just seems to lead further away from what we instinctively seek. Perhaps we are going in the wrong direction after all? Perhaps the external world can't give us peace? What if the carrot-on-the-stick of a pension or amassed possessions, doesn't actually give us what we really want, lasting satisfaction? What if, in all the striving and wanton squandering of our precious moments of calm, we arrive at the future-driven destination of retirement or a holiday or a mountain of gold, only to find that we've totally missed out on living? No wonder then that each 'achievement' has a hollow, empty ring to its applause. In your heart, in secret, the question arises: is that it?

In the midst of a pandemic, our world is going through lots of change which could be unsettling unless we learn from it. The drama of earthly incarnation is subject to constant change so do we remain ego-blinkered and bound to suffering or do we awaken to inner peace? Remember how peaceful it was during lockdown? The personal 'world' for each one of us shrank to our own four walls. No planes, no cars, no bustle, just quiet and unflustered simplicity of living. The calm was a perfect opportunity to retreat within, to step off the mortal treadmill for a while, an opportunity to rethink and to meditate. But we don't need to wait for a lockdown to find Inner Peace. We can commit to a daily 'lockdown', to go within, to tune into the one constancy: a profound peace, far beyond the perpetual flux of earthly living. Although this world appears at times to be chaotic, in meditation we discover that everything is unfolding perfectly for our spiritual awakening. Karma inexorably leads us to experience *exactly* what we need to learn to find that peace within.

Isn't it interesting that we all like stories? Did you know that every narrative boils down to one of only nine possible plot lines? Each fable may have different characters, different settings and goals but essentially there is an underlying commonality of seeking happiness by getting the bride, the castle, obtaining the prize, power, money etc. and having to overcome some obstacle in the search of that goal. Every good narrative will entertain at one level, of characters in a fictitious role set in the backdrop of a dramatic time or space where the hero or heroine has to overcome a great trial in order to find what they think will bring them peace and happiness. At one level, the reader may be simply seeking escapism from what assails them in their own personal dramas, a way of closing the blinds to the world and disappearing into someone else's plotline for a while. But at a far deeper level, the reader may, consciously or unconsciously, draw parallels with their own narrative playing out in their own battle of daily life, by way of seeking solutions to their own problems.

Life is a battlefield. Let's make no mistake about it: your narrative (parentage, childhood, environment), your character (name, status, zodiac sign, temperament), your plotline (actions, pitfalls, windfalls, achievements) and your personal quest for happiness (goals, dreams, aspirations), are all presented as an in-your-face reality and no matter how many times your choices lead you down a blind alley that doesn't result in happiness, the main character, you, can't seem to win. That's the game of life. Let me say, that if you thought the goal was out there in the maze of avenues and puzzle of choices, let me give you a shortcut: you're looking in the wrong direction.

The Bhagavad Gita (meaning 'song of the soul') is a scriptural depositary of highly practical wisdom, written by the sage Vyasa as a guide through the nitty-gritties of winning on the battlefield of life. The goal of finding lasting happiness and inner peace is achieved only when the soul becomes self-aware and realises the Self is One with the Great Oneness.

The battle of the soul to wrest back control from the wayward ego is waged on three main fronts: to respond with wisdom to events in the external world instead of reacting from ego-based habit; to respond with an inward-focused, even-minded stoicism to sensations from the senses instead of favouring pleasure and shunning pain or discomfort; to gain control of the mind (*manas*), will, and feelings (*chitta*) and go within in meditation, thereby finding your true self: the soul.

In the journey of becoming self-aware, the intrepid soul has to overcome all manner of ego attachments to worldly circumstances, such as, attachment to status afforded by birth, race, career, power or money. Slowly, the soul learns not to mistake what is only the subject of the narrative in their assigned role in the drama of life, with its true self. Eventually, the soul realises that all the blind alleys of the narrative are red herrings for they do not yield the lasting happiness that they promise. As long as the ego holds sway, then the self is continually bound to search the empty winding trails of the storyline of this lifetime and all other lifetimes to come. Until, the self starts to wonder if life is a charade: like being the star of its very own melodrama. As long as the vision is looking outwards into the drama, there is an alluring reality to it all: the bills are real; the enemies are real; the worries are real; pain is real! But eventually the self becomes tired of the drama and goes within for answers. That's when real life begins.

The second battle is to practise a healthy indifference to sensory feedback from the body. The ego is naturally a pleasure seeker and develops an aversion to pain or discomfort. The spiritual aspirant needs to overcome attachment to thoughtlessly reacting to the pairs of opposites presented to the senses: pleasure and pain; heat and cold. It is well known that a country child will feel pain less than a city kid as in the school of hard knocks, the pain register in the brain can be tuned down. Too much soft living without exposure to bodily discomforts just encourages over-sensitisation to sensation. It helps to tell yourself that it isn't cold or it doesn't hurt. It really works to immediately switch your attention elsewhere after a sharp bump, disallowing any yelp or blame reaction and pretend it hasn't happened (this can be so successful that sometimes I have only vague memory of where I obtained a bruise). The ego likes reaction. The soul wins by practising indifference.

The third type of battle is to go within in meditation. The ego is so used to having its own way, thinking whatever runaway thoughts it likes, kind or nasty, happy or wallowing in sadness. The ego thrives on attention and drama. When the soul tries to assert its natural dominance, the ego throws up a smokescreen of random thoughts designed to snare the inward-looking soul. This battle is challenged over micro-moments of time as each couple of seconds the ego throws up another distraction as if to say: look at this, isn't this more interesting than meditating? That battle can seem almost continuous from the moment that the eyes close and the self looks within, however, with practice more and more power over the will is in the soul's control. Eventually the soul, with the help of good-habit soldiers, will banish any interruptions from the screen of the mind and reassert its reign in the bodily kingdom.

So how do we start to move away from knee-jerk reactions

and practise even-mindedness? Whenever I had a problem which arose in daily life or found I'd reacted without thinking to the unkind words of others or environmental events, I would go within to meditate and be in the presence with my divine guru, Paramahansa Yogananda. In the quiet, I would ask for help. No matter what the issue was, for months in meditation, his inner prompting was always the same: look up. The level of the eyes gives a quick way of raising your focus from the drama to reality. That may seem too simple, but then the answer to all of life's mysteries *are* simple. It's the ego that makes things complicated. Looking up instantly raises the level of consciousness through which we are viewing life and gives us access to a higher state of consciousness.

The ego-self which looks out on the drama of life without looking in, only has access to the limited horizons of the conscious mind. The sub-conscious mind may filter through thoughts and feelings to the ego during sleep or day-dreaming as latent impressions of hidden fears and memories of a reality other than the everyday world, but the ego largely has little control over this. The wide perception of super-conscious awareness of the soul is not accessible to the ego-self. In meditation, the observer goes within and learns to wrest control from the ego (conscious and sub-conscious mind) and open the eyes of soul consciousness on the unlimited expansive vista seen by the super-conscious mind.

The level of the physical eyes is key to accessing the super-conscious mind: are you looking out from the level of the two physical eyes? Up? Down? Left to right? Raising the eyes by looking up to the level of the brow is a very quick way to raise your attunement to a higher vibrational state of awareness. On the brow between and slightly above the eyebrows is the *ajna* chakra: the centre of will. The power of will is accessed by turning the beam of the two physical eyes to this single point, the gateway to higher states of consciousness.

Imagine that there were many layers of vibration, like a pile of papers, stacked one on top of the other. The further you go down the pile of paper, the denser the experience is. You can learn to take your attention to successively higher and higher states of vibration, through the 'sheets of paper' (or veils of reality) until you leave behind manifested creation as an awakened being. A perfected being leaves behind limitation and attachment, for wondrous bliss, expansion and omnipresence.

Would that it were as simple as to climb up the layers of vibration to a happier state of being and stay there but latent karma from past lives accrued from the thoughts, words and deeds of this present incarnation, stored as seed tendencies (*samskaras*) and habits in the astral body, will keep pulling us down in vibration. I once heard spiritual progress described as 'three steps forwards, two steps back' and that pretty much sums up the experience: you achieve a higher vibration but the store house of karma pulls you back. At the same time life attracts to you fresh scenarios of opportunity to lay the past to rest. In my experience, this almost entirely involves letting go of attachment to fear/guilt/blame/anger etc. and coming to terms with the fact that it was the ego's choice to hold on to the kite strings of attachment realising it is the soul's choice to let go of the strings and give up that fight. As long as you hold on to 'fight', there will be no peace within.

In everyday life, you are learning to extricate yourself from whatever scenario may be playing out in the storyline of your life and to raise your vibration to a higher state of being to solve the predicament. A quick way to attune to a higher vibration is to look up. This takes you away from whatever is playing out in the narrative of your life. You can also mentally look up. This gives you space to step within and gives you the tools and the detachment to make an intelligent choice.

These are the tests of daily living, that you are not overcoming the issue itself but are overcoming your false self. In letting go of that attachment to feeling hurt or harmed from a frozen moment in time we can begin to realise that it is not the events themselves which define us but whether we are attached to the emotional response to that frozen moment. Why are some people traumatised by something and others aren't? It's attachment. So, do you live your life letting go or do you hold on, allowing defining moments to colour everything? Spiritually successful people know how to let go of the past. Specific events are just chapters in the revealing of who we really are, we don't limit our 'becoming'. In other words, we live life, we don't let defining moments live us.

In these pivotal moments that life throws to you, you are being handed an opportunity to change. You are not being dealt a bad hand of cards or thrown a curve ball by life. You are being offered a possibility of change and of finding a lasting solution. The solution may simply be to deal kindly with those in that pivotal moment. But it may be that you just need to walk away. What is important is that you remain calm and use the tools gained through your meditation practice: to let nothing ripple the ocean of your consciousness; to remain within the deep peace in the centre; and to maintain that state of being as you go about the challenges of daily life.

Some of the ego's attachments to habitual responses can be extremely subtle but with developed scrutiny, the keen eye of discernment recognises even the softest whisper of ego's interference by how it feels. The key signature of the ego is fear or feeling small and contracted. Remember that fear is just a vibration. The Self eventually weeds out each fear in meditation, revealing more and more of the light of the indwelling soul. Each moment is a fresh chance to gain mastery. With the eyes looking upward towards the brow you have access to the super-conscious level of awareness, and are no longer limited to ordinary everyday consciousness which only has access to limited mind. When you raise your awareness, you are no longer limited and you have access to a zillion possible solutions. One of those solutions may be just to walk away. The skirmish of consciousness is lost if you let the ego react. Know that you have the tools and strength of mind to remain unruffled in any situation life presents to you. You would not be having the experience unless it was well within your capability to overcome the inner battle.

As our world goes through enormous change, it becomes even more important to maintain your peace. We can learn to carry that peace as an untouchable state, carrying it preciously within us to all that we meet in our day to day lives. By meditating, we are ambassadors of peace and can affect hundreds of others in a positive and lasting way just by carrying that Peace within us. As Ambassadors of Peace, we are changing the world by carrying with us a harmonious inner calm which we share with each person that we meet.

* * *

This book is a treasure house of simple exercises distilling complex yoga philosophy into a pathway to assess and continually appraise spiritual progress inwards in the quest for inner peace. Through easy yoga breathing techniques, introspection and meditations on peace you can learn to overcome the reactionary ego and reveal who you are: the indwelling soul. Chapter by chapter we explore direct experiences of peace, firmly embedding the quality and lasting presence of peace in our lives.

How to Meditate

When learning to meditate, I like to keep things simple. Routine helps to prepare the body for sitting without fidgeting for a period of time. It can help to do things in a certain order, much like the sequence of events that you run through in getting ready for sleep. Although this shouldn't become monotonous or it may feel like a chore: spice things up sometimes by preparing in a different order.

My first experience of meditating in my teens was from a book by Barry Long. He wrote in bullet points, simple statements which appealed to me. So here is my simple in-a-nutshell guide:

- Do some physical stretching and breathing first with a focus on oxygenating the brain. It is easier to let the body sit quietly after it has been stimulated by gentle exercise and energised. Practise a few yoga asana postures if you know any. Alternatively, stand outside in the fresh air and breathe in deeply and fully, lifting the arms overhead and lowering as you exhale. Focus on releasing physical and mental 'static' and filling up with *prana* (life force) from the air.
- Be seated upright. It isn't important whether you sit in a chair or cross-legged, just be comfortable. The important consideration is that the spine is upright. This helps to keep you alert and present. The goal is to take the consciousness inward in meditation and an alert body posture guards against drifting off into the dreamy state of the subconscious or sleep.
- Sway from left to right a few times until your consciousness is centred in the spine. You can recognise that you are centred by the feeling of calm, like the eye of the storm: all of the restlessness is outside of the central column of the spine. Within the physical spine are the more subtle spines. The vital life force *(prana)* runs through the spine. In order to ascend to higher states of awareness in meditation, the spine must be straight. A sagging spine gives the message to the body to drift away from alertness.
- Pray. Praying in the language of your heart to God, Allah, Krishna, Jesus Christ, a guru or any saint creates a link

to that enlightened personage. Even if they are no longer in incarnation, they will place you in a direct beam of light lifting your consciousness and often blessing your spiritual practice, not only making it easier to go within but helping you to progress by releasing the ego's hold.

- Watch the breath. Remember: you are not this body. Watch the breath objectively, as if you were watching someone else breathing. Watching the breath helps withdraw awareness away from sensation on the skin towards the spine and brain. Watch little rivulets of life force flow back from the edges of the skin into the upward torrent in the spine.

- *So Ham* Mantra. Keep watching the breath. As the body breathes in, mentally say *So* (as in 'no'). As the body breathes out, mentally say *Ham* (as in 'ram'). The *So Ham* mantra means 'He I am' (or 'That I am') and reminds us that we are not the body or any external experience, we are the Great Spirit. This mantra is the vehicle of a subtle but very powerful shift in consciousness. Mentally chant it as if your soul were singing it.

- Swami Shankara stated that through the *So Ham* mantra, enlightenment can be achieved. After a while, the breath will be secondary to the mental mantra. Let the syllables resonate on the core of your being. Continue for 10–30 minutes.

- Listen attentively in the quiet. Listen from the space between the two ears as if you might miss something really important if you let your attention waver.

- The ego may throw up thought distractions into the quiet. Try to maintain looking up towards the brow chakra. Know that random thought impressions may percolate up from the peripheries but if you keep your attention on looking through the brow, any thought impressions bubble on past without interrupting your concentration.

Thought impressions cannot coalesce into reality if you don't give them your attention. They simply vaporise into nothingness. You are in charge. You have willpower over the ego. You can decide what you place your attention on.

The mind is difficult to control and restless; but, by practice and by dispassion it may be restrained!
Bhagavad Gita 6:35

Learn to school the unruly mind. Krishna extols Arjuna (who represents you as the Soul, in the journey of life) that the mind is fickle but it can be brought into control by yoga meditation and dispassion (not letting yourself be carried away by the mind). So in meditation, you are learning to control the mind. The same experience rarely comes up twice in a meditation, even if you are repeating the formula of a meditation because each day you are facing a new version of you. Remember, you are not this body, not the breath, not this mind, not the character and circumstances which you find yourself in. You are pure Soul and as such, you are training yourself to be in the moment of whatever arises. The more that you meditate, the more you identify with the soul with its keynote signature, bliss. In meditation, you are training yourself to remember and consciously attune to your true soul state of tranquillity.

As you sit down to meditate each day, you are showing up on the battlefield of life to face the ego as the foe of your natural soul tranquillity. The false-self's natural state is restlessness and it endeavours to keep you entranced by the world at large through perpetual feedback from the senses. That tug-of-war is ever present, whether you are consciously aware of it or not. In garnering your will to meditate, you face all manner of distractions on the battlefield with your ego self. You have your meditation tools as methods that work to override whatever restlessness arises in the mind or body.

We must be present in the moment when we meditate. I have found that seeking a specific result in meditation simply pushes it further away. One just has to do the practice and be in each moment as it arises. The pursuing of peace through the non-pursuing is a tricky concept to get your head around but suffice to say that this will become clearer over time should you simply show up in the moment with your full attention. You may have to root out over time any ego weeds holding on to a secret future agenda of attaining peace. That means that any thoughts of 'what may come next' is superseded in your consciousness with just experiencing the now. I state this point from the outset as it may dramatically benefit us, as the seeker, if we able to hold onto this concept before practice.

This simple practice is the starting place of any of the meditations in this book. It is a profound practice in itself and can take between 20 and 60 minutes a day, depending on your own circumstances.

It can be helpful to have a meditation space such as the same chair, a corner of a room or a meditation blanket, as the *prana* that you generate during meditation will gather there. This not only helps you develop a good habit but the vibration in your seat, corner or blanket can help facilitate the lift of your consciousness more quickly into a meditative state.

Sitting for meditation is always easier when the world is quiet. The ether is quietest in the dark of night as the restless thoughts of your household and neighbours are at rest then and so it is most conducive for meditation. Popular times to practise are early morning before breakfast, and just before or three hours after the evening meal. As we withdraw attention within in meditation, we seek to drop physical awareness and tune upward into the extremely subtle vibration of peace. A heavy meal is counterproductive to this goal as the physical body's resources are downward focused on digestion which often leads to drowsiness. One must be alert and present.

Finally, it is helpful to know that it is your soul destiny to succeed in achieving liberation over the ego-self which is blind to all the subtle wonders that await you in spiritual enlightenment. Follow your soul-longing and meditation will set you free.

With all my blessings of peace and love,
Jenny Light

Peace flows through my heart, and blows through me
as a zephyr.
Peace fills me like a fragrance.
Peace runs through me like rays.
Peace stabs the heart of noise and worries.
Peace burns through my disquietude.
Peace, like a globe of fire, expands and fills my omnipresence.
Peace, like an ocean, rolls on in all space.
Peace, like red blood, vitalizes the veins of my thoughts.
Peacelike a boundless aureole, encircles my body of infinity.
Peace-flames blow through the pores of my flesh, and through
all space.
The perfume of peace flows over the gardens of blossoms.
The wine of peace runs perpetually through the winepress of
all hearts.
Peace is the breath of stones, stars, and sages.
Peace is the ambrosial wine of Spirit flowing from the cask of
silence,
Which I quaff with my countless mouths of atoms.
Metaphysical Meditations, Paramahansa Yogananda

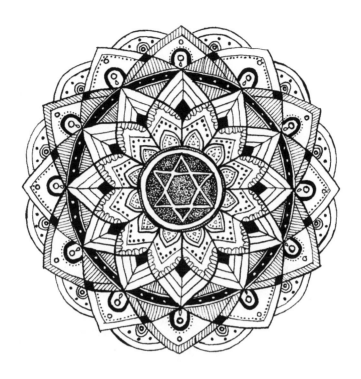

Chapter 1

Peace Is Always Present

In this world of constant change, peace often seems to be an elusive quality. Nothing sits still. Nothing is immune to decay before the process of renewal to be reborn in another guise or phase of life. Everything in the physical world is subject to change: civilisations rise and diminish; bodies are born and die in the cycle of life; the seasons and tides are perpetually in motion; even our own breath is never at peace. Nothing in the physical world remains constant. From fear born of lack of security due to this perpetual flux, we attempt to bring stability and insurance of a buffer against the results of constant change. We build walls within and without with the misguided notion that we can stem the flow of change. It's as futile as the legendary King Canute demanding the tide to cease. In building walls to halt change, we shut out the subtle flow of peace itself.

You might wonder where peace is in an existence where nothing stands still. Is peace an impossible dream or an achievable reality? What if that peace which you are seeking is already flowing through you right now? What if the inner clamour and mental agitation are drowning out the quiet soothing constant voice of peace? If so, how do we tune out one and amplify the other?

In this chapter, we explore a method of retuning the dial of our inner experience to the gentle flow of perpetual peace and to find a calm endurance to chart the ship of consciousness through calm or stormy seas with equal even-mindedness. *Titiksha*, a Sanskrit term meaning 'calm endurance', is the trademark of a true yogi: to be able to weather choppy waves of experience without being disturbed by the changes that occur. *Titiksha* is fostered by holding an objective calmness to endure whatever circumstances arise and meditation is the method of developing that objective calmness of body, mind and spirit. The trials and tribulations of everyday circumstances give us the training ground of opportunities in which to practise responding with that calm evenness of mind to a gamut of mildly annoying to supremely challenging experiences. Until you have mastered *titiksha*, the gentle flow of inner peace will elude you.

Peace is the true nature of God and our true state of being. Until we make the shift in consciousness through meditation, we simply don't realise that. Until we wake up to how we are operating in this world, we are constantly filtering our experiences through three alternating modes of experience:

Excitable happiness in response to pleasurable circumstances.

Morose unhappiness in reaction to unpleasant circumstances.

A flat-line of indifference or boredom between these periods of happiness and unhappiness.

None of these modes are a state of 'being at peace'. These are agitated peaks and troughs of the waves of life when operating through ego consciousness. They are a veil covering the true soul state of perpetual calm and the deeper state of peace which lies beneath them. Meditation is the process by which we pull back that veil and gradually the eyes of soul-perception reveal your true nature beneath the perpetually agitated ego consciousness. None of these three modes is your true state of being. Perhaps you are aware that you are using the restlessly active energy of the heart to operate every thought or action through one of these modes.

I first became aware of these three disquieting modes as a recurring pattern in how I was living my life to seek acclaim from others or in trying to avoid boredom when I burned myself out in my forties. In my first book, *Living Lightly: A Journey through Chronic Fatigue Syndrome (M.E.)*, Ayni Books, 2016, I describe how I would avoid boredom at all costs, challenging myself to beat time by filling each waking moment with some task or other professionally, creatively or in household chores. I was so ego-bound that I foolishly took pride in how productive I was but as a result I was never at peace within. I had made agitation my bedfellow and it ultimately burned me out. Never to lie down to a challenge, even when lying prone for hours a day as forced by my health, I saw this too as a challenge. I viewed my health crisis with the eyes of reason and I set my will to get well and utilise 30 years of experience in meditation to calm those restless waves within. The three modes of excitable happiness in pursuit of some external goal, unhappiness at the thwarting of my ego goals or boredom at having nothing physical to do, all came into stark focus for what they were: a revealing of the restless ego within. My mind was like a caged animal pacing up and down, never at peace, ceaselessly looking for distraction after distraction from going within. I realised how errant my mind really was and saw this as a real opportunity to find myself.

There was literally no running away from the experience. The agitation of my ego consciousness was like painful jagged lines running through me and I was forced (or guided) by my soul to slowly extricate myself from that ego-bound habitual modality to find the calmness behind those three states of restlessness.

Calmness is the forerunner to actual experience of peace. Peace is the only true constant. Everything else is just passing clouds on the screen of the script for this incarnation. Meditation will open the eyes of your awareness to reveal that you are not helplessly bobbing on the disquieting waves of excitable happiness, morose unhappiness and boredom or indifference, tossed like a piece of flotsam on the sea of life at the mercy of the run-away ego's reactionary emotional states. You had simply allowed that 'reality' to be how you operated your life. Meditation allows you to access the wisdom of the soul and to envisage operating your life through the sweetness of the soul as an altogether more peaceful experience. But this takes practice.

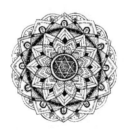

Exercise: Observation of My Habitual Mode of Being

Sit upright. Become aware of the regularity of the breathing. Allow the exhale to be longer than the inhale.

Tune into the heart area. Sit quietly for a few moments focusing on long slow breaths and the process of breathing.

Ask yourself: Am I fully engaged in observing the breath or is part of my awareness holding back?

Which of these three states am I filtering my life through, if any?

How am I habitually filtering my life through the heart?

Am I holding on to any heaviness in the heart as sorrow, excitable emotions or a state of boredom?

Am I fluctuating between these states of being?

Do I *like* being restless? Do I have reservations about being fully conscious of being peace?

How much of my consciousness is invested in restlessness? Does it make me feel like I'm in control?

Do I feel like a cork bobbing helplessly on the ocean of circumstance?

How much am I aware of my soul as being as deep and peaceful as the whole ocean?

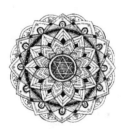

Use your observation as a guide to change your habitual modes of being where you allow yourself to filter your experience in reaction to that which is happening around you. Your aim is to be able to hold on to calm even-mindedness and to weather the choppy waves of experience without being disturbed by what occurs in whatever part you are called upon to play in this earthly incarnation.

Restless wandering thoughts must be controlled and calmed in order to tune our consciousness to the sweet balm of peace. That Divine Peace is constantly flowing through you from God and the divine realm. The masters are beaming that peace to you, silently encouraging you to turn away from the distractions of the earthly playground and to find that Peace which already exists within.

By going within in meditation, we learn to hone our concentration to a single focus and to ignore valiantly the myriad of distractions from the senses and the wandering mind. The single focus in yoga practice is to place all your consciousness on an aspect of the divine as God, as the omnipotent Father, the tenderly loving Divine Mother, Buddha, Krishna, Jesus Christ, guru, a saint or any aspect that appeals to the yearning in your heart, most personally accessible for you. For all beings who have achieved *kaivalya* (soul liberation) there is no partiality, since they have fully realised their Great Oneness. It is important to hold in your mind's eye that aspect of the divine when you attempt to meditate as then you will not be meditating alone. By tuning into their holy vibration, they will guide your progress. Closing the eyes, we withdraw mental tendrils of distraction from all that can be felt, heard, smelled, seen or tasted, and to place that attention on your chosen aspect of the Divine.

In the beginning, extricating the mind from the messages of the senses is not easy so do not be discouraged. Yoga breath technique is a distinct aid in amplifying your efforts to keeping the mind 'on track'. Practice of breath techniques is invaluable in learning to face whatever arises in your meditation practice with a calm even-minded *titiksha*.

Lasting happiness is achieved by tuning into and maintaining an evenly peaceful state of mind. Learning objectively to watch the body breathing is vital to mastery of the body-mind. It sounds easy but how many times in the space of one minute will the ego attempt to drag the attention away on the lure of a distraction? Even harder to master is to simply watch the process of the body inhaling and exhaling without the ego seizing control of the observation process by manipulating when the breath starts and stops. Watching the breath sounds easy, but it isn't. What you often find is that it is the ego that you are watching, in all its wiles and power-seeking ways. If you find that a minute has gone by fruitlessly, don't get annoyed with yourself (that is one of the ego's ploys) but just patiently keep releasing the errant attention. Place it back on watching the inhale and simply watching the exhale to the last expulsion of air.

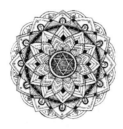

Exercise: Watching the Breath

Allow the breath to become still. Tune into the spine as an upright rod of light.

Visualise the lungs either side of the spine. Objectively watch the process of breathing in and out, almost as if you were watching someone else breathing.

Notice the change in temperature of the breath: cool with the inhale and warmer with the exhale.

Realise that your body which you are observing breathing is not you (for in truth this body is not you). It has a soft inhale and soft exhale.

Try to just observe without letting the ego consciousness step in and anticipate the next breath or the next part of the breath cycle. Just observe.

Try to be with the process of the inhale, without anticipating the exhale.

Sometimes it is useful to just listen to the sound of the breath in the throat or the sensation. This could be the sensation of coolness or warmth as it passes through the throat.

If the ego tries to interject, just quietly extricate your awareness and place it gently back on just observing. Repeat for 5 minutes.

Mastering objectivity in watching the breath is pivotal to your spiritual progress. Be aware that the ego will find this boring, but resolve to sit for the full five minutes at every practice. Be a spiritual scientist: put the breathing process under the scrutiny of the keen eyes of the soul. Ignore all the distractions of the wandering ego-led mind. Experiment with how detached you can become from the physical process of breathing. Remind yourself: 'I am not the body. The body is breathing. I am merely watching the mechanical process of its inhale and exhale. I am not the breath.'

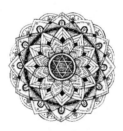

It is God's dearest wish that you turn away from all the toys that He has provided you with and return to your home in spirit. Your soul is everlasting and eternal but you are bound to return to earth in repeated incarnations until you fully realise your true state. In other words, until you awaken to who you *really* are, you will be bound to return to earth in a future physical body until you rise above the human condition.

Practise an inward even-minded smile to all of the events of the narrative of this incarnation. Each day gives you a fresh slate to perfect your practice of *titiksha*. Let nothing ruffle your feathers: each circumstance is sent, not to try you, but as a gentle prod to remind you to awaken from the cosmic slumber of this world. Never forget that this is not your true home: that glorious heavenly state of being awaits those who have mastered even-mindedness. Next time that you find a wave of irritation or agitation washing over you, rein it in. Release it to the wind with a little private smile *God is with me and reminding me to not be disturbed by this. I am spirit.* Pray silently for aid in quietening the internal storm in the language of your soul. Mentally chanting the *So Ham* mantra in moments of trial is very calming and creates a soothing balm on rippled waters of spirit. *So Ham*, meaning 'He I am', subtly reminds you not to identify with the role you are playing in this earthly *lila* (Divine play).

Maya, the great illusion, is so entrancing. You only have to observe the instinctive behaviour of people in gloomy or rainy weather scurrying around looking down as if somehow to avert getting wet. A recoiled protective gesture tells the body that there is something to be afraid of and the mood is thereby likely to be gloomy too. In Scotland the weather is so wet and changeable that it gives plenty of lessons on developing a yogic indifference to cold, hot, wet or sunshine! To develop a healthy stoicism, it is helpful to remember that the rain will descend whether you cower or walk with your head held high. As an act of mindfulness, you could decide to enjoy the refreshing smell of plants in the rain or enjoy the cool sensation of the rain on your face. Attitude is everything. In both scenarios, the rain still falls but in one there is a perception of suffering and in the other, a placing of consciousness in a state of dispassion (*tikisha*) or an attached in-the-moment enjoyment. We can enjoy that which we must endure. A state of even-mindedness to endure that which we cannot change is a vital lesson in rising above the illusion.

The secret in spiritual advancement is to be non-reactive to anything that life can throw at you: bodily discomfort, pain, mental suffering or anger that comes your way. Be mentally detached from the situation and try to enjoy it objectively. You can convert all circumstances to happy ones if you change your mental focus. That is where your meditation practice comes to your aid: it gives you an inner experience of peacefulness, which will help foster even-mindedness in all circumstances. Don't just take my word for it! This is scientifically proven:

meditate and you will be surprised how things that used to irk you no longer have any hold over you. You can see them for what they are, just a valuable opportunity to illustrate to you that you are not the drama. You learn to stop fostering a belief in separateness by holding on to these three false modes of being. Anything that arises in reaction to external circumstances is false. Circumstances come and go. Accept them as you would a dream. Nothing can harm you. They constantly change, but you, the soul, are changeless and in constant peaceful ever-new bliss. You are not helpless, as a cork bobbing directionless on the ocean of circumstance. You, the soul, have a chance to awaken through whatever happens to be playing out on the script of your life and to play it out with an inner happiness.

There is a discrimination to be made here between the ego's reactionary 'happiness' which is in response to that which you deem to be pleasurable, and to that innate soul happiness which is happy for its own sake. Soul happiness could be experienced even in the direst circumstances. I recall an earlier difficult period in my own life when my first marriage was breaking up; even though I seemed to be playing out a disassociated state towards the object of his anger, I no longer had any desire to participate in the habitual retorts. Even in the heat of the moment, I found myself feeling compassion for another soul who was still snared by his ego, sending him love and blessing after blessing. I realised there and then that anger could not harm me. I felt happy. It was literally like awakening from a dream of eons. Meditation had given me a healthy objectivity and the tools to maintain being in that deep soul-happiness even when I wasn't sitting in meditation. I could have felt unhappy but I didn't: that was only the story that was playing out at that time.

Meditation after meditation we are peeling back layer after layer of the ego. Bit by bit we are finding out: what is me, the soul? And what is the ego? The ego has many wiles but you learn to peel back to find out who you are in all of this.

If you are not experiencing peace all the time, it is because you are attached to replaying a habitual programme of sadness, happiness or indifference as a result of what appears to be happening in the drama or circumstances in which you find yourself. While tossed on stormy seas of illness, times of physical endurance or emotionally charged moments when everything seems to be going wrong and the world is falling down around you, I find it very helpful to remind myself during challenging circumstances, that that moment is gone. If there is another wave of suffering that comes up, again mentally repeat *this too shall pass*. You learn not to engage with the suffering or the perception that there is suffering. There is a perception of suffering if you tune into it, placing it full-frontal in your awareness, but you can choose not to engage with suffering. Each time that you engage with enduring the moment through the affirmation *this too shall pass*, that moment is conquered. Life is a series of moments which constitute one day. Each day is a fresh start and you have blissful sleep in between. In sleep you are not engaged with this world: you are in a subconscious or super-conscious state in the astral world, and each morning you awaken to take up your earthly role once more in a fresh new day filled with many potential opportunities to become soul aware.

Meditation builds the mental stamina and objective strength of will to rise above waves of restless agitation, fear or annoyance. In those moments, keep reminding yourself:

This experience shall pass. I am not this body for I have been many bodies before. I am not this mind for only the intuitive perception of my soul can see beyond this physical smokescreen of illusion. Everything is helping me to evolve spiritually. I am calm. I am peaceful.

Since you are reading this book, you are likely to have begun the journey of soul awakening into your true soul awareness of being in peaceful, blissful oneness, *irrespective of whatever is playing out in the external role of this life.* You are not this body: the body changes but your soul is changeless. You are not this character or role in life: these merely present a convenient learning opportunity for your soul growth. At the end of earthly life, you are essentially the same: untouched by any experience. You, the soul, can never be hurt and has never been hurt: it's only a perception of false self (the ego) that you have been harmed by any events in the script of an incarnation.

The Self cannot be cut, burnt, wetted nor dried up. It is eternal, all-pervading, stable, ancient and immovable.
Bhagavad Gita 2:24

Awakening to expansive soul peacefulness means that you still continue to act in this world and fulfil your God-given role but you realise that *how* you respond is imperative to soul awakening. If you are not experiencing peace, it is because the ego is presenting a barrier through one of the three reactionary states of restlessness: excitable happiness, sadness or boredom. Inner peace will be revealed once you learn to quell these disquieting waves.

Your job is to meditate to develop and refine body, mind and spirit and to consciously weed out the ego's impediments as these are revealed to you.

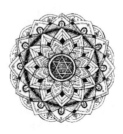

In the Moon of Peace Meditation, we are learning to still the waves of restlessness through bringing the hands together in *namaste* at the heart. During the busyness of the day, the life force is dissipated into multitudinous tasks through activity with the hands. In this meditation, we are consciously surrendering the life force from each hand to flow into the other, effectively allowing the outwardly-dissipated life force and consciousness to reverse its current and be retained within the body. As we bring the hands together, we gather awareness from the external environment and the surface of the skin to flow into the heart area. This meditation uses a focus on the light of the moon, which is the symbol of the soul. We cannot see true self unless seen with the clear reflected light of the soul. When deeply focused in meditation the soul sees a pure reflection of itself on the brow, as a shining disc of light, at the spiritual eye (*ajna chakra*).

Moon of Peace Meditation

Sit upright and gently close the eyes.

Bring the palms together in praying hands at the heart. Become aware of the balance of being in the centre as the life force from the left palm flows into the right palm and the life force in the right palm flows into the left.

Prayer: *Divine Father, awaken my heart to Thy flow of peace. Awaken my soul in Thy Oneness and peace. Help me to move through the distractions in life with an even-minded heart, awake and aware in Thy consciousness. Om Shanti, Peace.*

Let the hands rest on the thighs. Breathe in deeply through the nostrils and exhale through an open mouth with an elongated sigh, letting go of all tension in the body. Repeat twice more, breathing away all clouds from the mind as well as the body.

Practise Watching the Breath until the mind becomes calm (5 minutes).

Pivot your eyes under the closed lids towards the *ajna* chakra (between the eyebrows) without straining. Imagine that you are breathing in through the brow as if it were a great light like a full moon.

Breathe in and out a long, smooth breath through that great light on the brow (as if it were a nostril).

Allow the current and focus of the two physical eyes to flow up into that great light on the brow.

Imagine that you are watching a reflection of the moon on a bowl of water. You can see the pure and calm reflection of the moon on the surface of the water.

If you were to blow on the water, it would break up the reflection into ripples on the surface. The alternating waves of experience (happiness, unhappiness or boredom) all create ripples on that perfect surface. Allow your breath to be so calm and focused that there is a perfect reflection of the moon in that basin of water.

As the body breathes slowly and smoothly, you can maintain focus on the perfect reflection of the moon on the surface of the water. The moon is the symbol of the soul. By calming the alternating waves of experience that the ego reacts to, we come back into the constant peace of the soul.

Breathe in smoothly and calmly.

Breathe out smoothly and calmly so that you maintain the perfect reflection of the moon on the water. Allow the flow of peace from the mooned face of your soul to flow through.

Mentally repeat this mantra:

Peace flows through my soul. Peace is always present.
I am held in Peace. Peace flows through my entire being.
I am buoyant in Peace. Peace is my essential nature.
I am nurtured in Peace. The ego may present many guises but still
I am sustained in Peace.

Imagine that you are basking in the mooned reflection of your soul, awake in perpetual peace.

Let go of the heaviness of the breath and experience peace in the pauses between inhale and exhale, exhale and inhale.

Mentally repeat as a mantra:

I am the flow of peace.

My peace abounds, flowing endlessly from the cup of spirit in my heart, spilling out from the boundaries of body, breath and mind and into an endless sea of peace.

I am no longer held prisoner by the ego.

I am the ever-expanding ocean of peace itself. I become the mooned light of my soul.

Peace flows perpetually from my overflowing heart.

Come back into awareness of the body. Visualise peace flowing into the cells of the body, filling each cell, breaking free of the bounds of each cell and spilling into the neighbouring cells. Visualise the whole body glowing in the experience of peace.

Take three full breaths in and out and come back into body consciousness.

Om Shanti Peace.

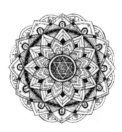

Try to maintain this walking, waking modality of peace for as long as you can throughout your day.

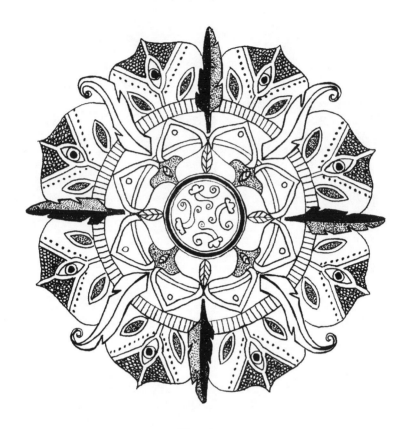

Chapter 2

Peace as the Softest Breeze

Peace comes as an otherworldly waft of a cool breeze on a hot day, like a cool refreshing drink quenching our soul-parched consciousness. How many times do we feel as dense and heavy as a sod of earth? This body of bones, sensation and skin is taxing on so many levels. The soft breeze of peace is a reminder from our soul of our true heritage, a siren call to 'wake-up!'

In this chapter, we are developing a perception of the softest subtle perception of peace through use of *pranayama* (breathing techniques) and continue to master *titiksha* by aiming to eliminate restless waves of reaction to pairs of opposites: heat and cold; pleasure and pain. As creatures of habit, we are accustomed to giving the ego operation of the gross body and mind in response to external stimuli. Like a donkey desirous of the dangled carrot, the ego is attracted to sense satisfactions which have resulted in a sensation of pleasure in past experiences, and avoiding circumstances which may result in pain or discomfort. In order to divest the ego from its slavery to attraction/repulsion, and wrest back control, we learn to restrain the body and mind from sensation by training the breath. Pranayama (life force control) techniques are highly effective for not only controlling the blind sense-led ego, but in purifying and elevating our consciousness to attune us to more subtle realms of being.

The senses are continually sending messages from the sense of touch to the brain as electrical signals. The nerves carry messages as a series of distinct electrical impulses which the brain then interprets as heat, cold, pleasure or pain. So it would be fair to say that, until the brain has deciphered the message, until that point the 'message' is just a report on a sensation. Whether the interpretation of the initial message is deemed as pleasant or unpleasant, the brain directs the body to react accordingly.

On the path of yoga, we learn to rise above all these pairs of opposites. We can learn to master the will to tell our body that it is not cold or it is not hot. These are just perceptions, an interpretation of like or dislike in response to a particular stimulus. One should, of course, employ common sense to not expose oneself to extremes of heat or cold which may cause the body temple injury. The physical body is our vehicle for this incarnation and should be cared for as one would a motor car if we expect it to convey us flawlessly from A to B: keep it clean, lubricated, well maintained and topped up with quality fuel. Moreover, this body temple temporarily houses our soul so that it learns the lessons of this incarnation and should be cared for as it is easier to fly high in our meditation from a healthy, well-functioning body than one which is experiencing pain or suffering.

The key point in catering for the needs of the physical body is to give the body its due attention but without becoming a slave to its sensory demands of avoidance of discomfort. The goal is to detach mentally from the body while at the same time seek to promote its healthy functioning and a suitable solution for any ailments. Give the body its place but without allowing it to dominate every waking moment of your thoughts. Therein lies the trap of earth-bound incarnation and bemiring in *maya*, the cosmic delusion. We should try to make this incarnation count for our spiritual progress and in order to do that we need to rise above body consciousness. Learning to mentally override sensations and restless thoughts are the battles that one has with the ego as we go within in meditation.

The self-controlled man, moving amongst objects with the senses under restraint, and free from attraction and repulsion, attains to peace.
Bhagavad Gita 2:64

When we can meditate without being disturbed by the senses, we find a deepening calm arising from within. The goal is to be unmoved by the messages, the perceptions, that the brain receives from the senses and to learn to mentally pull out the 'phone cable' of those sensations so that your meditation will not be disturbed for a while. We all know only too well that as we sit to meditate with the best of intentions that those are the times that Aunt Mary or a colleague might call us on the phone. Just as it is good practice to mute your phone or disconnect the wire before meditation, so it is in going within; we also mentally disconnect the wires from relaying a constant stream of messages from the surface of the skin, or from the other sense messages of smell, sight, hearing and taste.

Practising Disassociation from the Senses

There are two main points in practising disassociation from the senses. The first is endurance to changes of temperature, physical discomfort or pain as an act of will while acting in the world. The second is disassociation from the feedback of messages from the senses while practising meditation.

Endurance of Temperature, Discomfort or Pain in Daily Life

One can endure the discomfort of fluctuations of temperature or perception of pain without being disturbed by these changes. We can learn to ignore such discomforts with an even-mindedness. In the moment that you are receiving the sensation as a perception in the brain, know that it is only the physical body that is experiencing that discomfort.

For instance, on stubbing a toe on a coffee table that just seems to have got in our way, there is a brief moment when there is no pain, just awareness of impact. We know from experience that there is a delay in the sensation of pain before it washes over us with a sharp, but blessedly short-lived agony. In the relay of the messages from toe to brain, sensation arrives first and there is an infinitesimal delay before the pain receptors refer their message to the brain. This brief millisecond is our opportunity to practise endurance: to redirect our attention elsewhere until the flash of pain reverts to a sensation of heat before finally dissipating. Perhaps you can learn to walk away and ignore the impact, ignore the messages and continue toward your initial destination. Certainly do try to resist or over-ride any urge to retaliate or blame another for placing the object in your path. Just note if this is a pattern of reaction to injury for you and resolve to change it. I find it very helpful to immediately focus on breathing long, steady breaths and practise a mantra or think of my guru or a saint, and smile in that brief moment, trying to act as they would.

The point is that you have a choice in how you respond to an injury, heat or cold. To be mentally and emotionally unruffled by the experience of discomforting sensations takes practice. Don't beat yourself up if you observe that you are reacting, either outwardly or inwardly, just practise patiently disengaging your consciousness. As many times as it takes, patiently place your attention elsewhere. Life will throw up lots of chances to practise unruffled-ness until you can master the lesson of endurance.

Disengagement from Sensation for Meditation

In meditation, mentally disengage from any fluctuating sensations. Imagine the body as a fine network of nerves from the surface of the skin, feeding into larger neural pathways leading to the mainframe computer: the brain. In receiving messages from the outer edges of its awareness, the brain prioritises its response on a scale of merely annoying, such as an itch, to those that are potentially life threatening. Obviously, we should allow appropriate movement that will take the physical body out of danger from harm but it is those niggly urges to scratch or move which we can focus on ignoring as they are counterproductive to meditation.

As an example, you sit down to meditate with all the best of intentions, taking time to ensure that you are sitting upright in meditation posture. It is all going great for the first few minutes and then an urge to shift position arises. The awareness may be that the seat isn't comfy or a leg feels awkward or your clothing feels irritating. A practised meditator knows that this is just the initial stage of withdrawing awareness from the extremities of the body (*pratyahara*) and they know how to quickly bypass this stage by using techniques.

It is helpful to think of sensation as simply a message that is being perceived by the brain. But in the battlefield of meditation, the ego attempts to utilise all bodily sensation to try and lure the attention of any unsuspecting meditator into this trap of paying heed to these body messages until you realise that twenty minutes have gone by when all you have focused on *is* that urge to move. In that experience there is no calm. So, we go into meditation with a strong will to be prepared to sit still, no matter what sensation arises, and to re-route our attention on a breathing technique. Will changes thought into energy, giving us the strength of mind to overcome the pitfalls of ego consciousness.

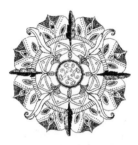

The following exercise helps you practise the first stage in withdrawing awareness from the body. The first shift in consciousness is to master pulling back energy from limbs and soft tissues to flow into the astral spine. You might think of yourself as a tree in the autumn pulling back its vital resources from the leaves as it prepares to shed its canopy.

Exercise: Withdrawing Awareness from the Edges of the Skin

Sit upright for meditation. Take a few minutes to watch the inhale and exhale as the breath transitions into longer, slower breaths.

Visualise the brain as a vast reservoir of light, receiving sensations as messages from the physical nerves and constant communications from the astral body of light. The brain is processing a huge amount of data every second as electrical messages from the physical body and as feelings from the astral body.

Visualise power from the astral body flowing down into the dense physical brain and into the spine. From the spine, power or *prana* flows in an outward current to every cell of the body.

Feel into the surface of the skin. What messages is the body relaying to the brain just now? Try to observe sensation objectively, as if you were a scientist remotely viewing the process.

Next, imagine that the surface sensation is just energy: a tingling ripple of *prana* (life force) as a sheet of energy over the whole body.

Visualise crystalline energy peeling back from the extremities of the legs and arms to empty into the *prana* tube of the spine.

Watch the shining tube of *prana* in the spine and head. Observe any movement of *prana* as the body inhales or exhales.

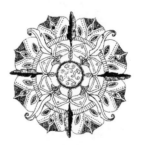

In developing even-mindedness and to cope with the extremes of summer heat, the *sheetali/sheetkari* breath practice is very effective. These are tranquilising *pranayamas* which cool the system and withdraw the awareness away from the physical body. These techniques have essentially the same effect, breathing long and slow through the mouth. *Sheetali* is for those who can roll their tongue and *sheetkari* is for those who cannot roll their tongue. They are an excellent preparation for meditation or they can be used as standalone 'first aid' techniques. I have also found them useful in cooling menopausal flushes!

Pranayama Technique for Managing Heat: *Sheetali* or *Sheetkari* Breath

Sit upright in a relaxed but alert posture. Close the eyes. Take a deep breath in and sigh out in a long exhalation through an open mouth, mentally releasing mental and physical restlessness. Repeat three times.

Let the breath return to normal. Observe the temperature of the inhale and exhale.

Roll the sides of the tongue so that it forms a tube (*sheetali*) or close the teeth together and pull back the lips to expose the teeth (*sheetkari*). Breathe in a long slow breath through the tongue tube or through the closed teeth over a flat tongue. As you breathe in, slightly tip the chin towards the ceiling. There should be a sucking sound accompanied with an icy cold sensation on the tongue and roof of the mouth.

At the end of the inhalation, close the lips and touch the tongue to the roof of the mouth.

Breathe out through the nose and return the chin to level. Mentally hold on to the experience of coolness as you exhale.

Aim to develop experiencing cold on the tongue, throat and soft palette. Mentally think 'coolness' with each breath. Repeat for 12 breaths.

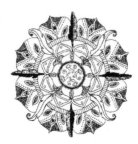

The aim of *sheetali/sheetkari pranayama* is to eliminate pairs of opposites that contribute towards restlessness. After this practice, seek to retain 'coolness' as a state of mind in the body and 'calmness' in the mind. We learn to eliminate concern for heat and can learn to take our attention out of the situation. When we become consumed with a perceived problem, we blow it out of proportion because that on which we focus is intensified.

Whatever you focus on increases.

Remember that as sparks of God-stuff, we have been given the power to manifest our immediate reality through our thoughts and words. As we progress on the spiritual path, we build the capacitor of the physical and astral bodies to hold greater and greater power or *prana* (life force). With this powerhouse comes an ever increasing onus to be mindful of what we are manifesting in that great beam of *prana*. We learn that to focus on the perceived stress, pain or suffering of the body, only amplifies it tenfold. We learn to refocus our perception on to peace and wellbeing within and without. It's all about our perception. You have the power to either believe that you are suffering or to understand that it's only a perception of suffering. Realise that you have a choice of where you place your attention.

An example of a change in perception:

I am suffering with toothache – the body experiences toothache, I perceive that I am well.

I'd like to share an exercise which I discovered while away on holiday when I experienced toothache. There was no access to a dentist so I went within in meditation to seek a solution. The following technique came to me and it utilises the pituitary gland as the master controller of the physical functions. My jaw was instantly numb. It gives pretty instantaneous natural pain relief.

Exercise for Coping with Pain

Take a deep breath in and sigh out to clear the mental screen.

Visualise your etheric 'hand' reaching in through the back of the head to cup the pituitary gland in the centre of the head. (Don't worry if your knowledge of anatomy isn't great. Just intending to connect with the pituitary gland will affect the same result. I imagined a little plum-shaped protrusion suspending from the brain.)

Imagine that you can feel it in your 'hand'. Mentally gently squeeze the pituitary with the intention of releasing the body's natural anaesthetic. Hold for one second. Release your 'hold' slightly and mentally direct the stream of pain-killing hormone to the affected area, left or right.

Repeat as necessary.

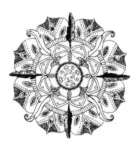

In this meditation, we move into the practice of observing that which is beneath the breath, symbolised by calming ego-rippled waters.

Meditation: Calm the Restless Waves of the Mind

Sit upright with the chin level. Take a deep breath in and sigh out three times, exerting the willpower to blow all restlessness out of the body, mind and spirit.

Prayer: *Divine Father, calm the storm of my restlessness and still the incessant ripples of the wave of my life. Reveal the ruffled face of Thy peaceful stillness, here and everywhere. Om Shanti Peace.*

Practise the *sheetali/sheetkari* breath for 12 rounds. Slow your practice right down so that you do not miss the elusive wisp of peace. If the mind starts to wander, rein it back in. Bit by bit you learn to quell the restless waves of the mind. Retain the cool calmness.

Let the breath return to its normal rhythm. Observe the body breathing.

Practise the mental mantra *So Ham*: as the body starts the in-breath, mentally say *So* and mentally say *Ham* as the body breathes out.

Try to extricate ego involvement with the *So Ham* mantra. Just observe the body breathing. Take control away from the breath so that it is a natural breath. Transfer your awareness to the mantra.

Allow the body to breathe as it will. The body may have periods when it wants to have pauses after the inhale or exhale, when we start to move into a 'breathless state'. Simply allow these pauses to arise.

Experience that mental repetition of *So* brings a cool breeze over the brain. *Ham* brings a cool breeze over the mind. Learn to let go so that the softness of the breeze passes through you.

Density falls away and you feel the lightness of the air.

Visualise how the soft quality of the breath is like the soft caress of an angelic hand. The air carries with it a gentle caress soothing over the consciousness of the mind and smoothing over the waters of the soul.

Imagine that you are insubstantial as if floating like a feather, elevating you to a higher state of being.

Allow the mantra to recede as you let go of the breath. Listen deeply within for the softest sound.

Perhaps there is the sound of a gentle wind through the trees or a gentle breeze from the sea rustling grasses. Perhaps there is the sound of soft music like a flute, played by the Divine Mother as a call to spirit. *Awaken! Come home to quiet everlasting peace in your true homeland of Spirit. There is only a dream of restlessness of earthly life. Your true state of being is one of everlasting peace.*

Allow the soft vibration of peace through the softest quality of air or as air blown through a flute. Experience a deeper relationship with Peace as it bubbles up from the depths quelling all waves of restlessness.

Imagine an angelic hand soothing the strings of your being. Remind yourself to not take life so seriously. This deeper experience with peace is who you really are: more precious than all the diamonds, gold or baubles of earthly life.

Let that softest of breezes blow through the wind of the mind. Visualise or perceive that it comes as a blessing directly from the Great Halls of Spirit.

Visualise the reflection of the full moon on a pot of water. When the surface is distorted, the reflection refracts into a thousand shards of light. When the surface becomes calm, the full light of the moon is reflected on the surface of the water.

Let go of more and more bodily identification or distraction by the mind. Whatever is perceived or presented, let go of that in your attention. Patiently keep extricating the awareness and placing it on the perception of calmness.

Perhaps there is awareness of perpetual peace deep beneath the waters of the mind, untouched by the comings and goings on the surface.

Imagine or experience the softest of breezes blowing over the surface of the mind as if blowing across a sheet of glass.

Peace extends to the further most reaches of awareness to the perimeters of perception. It flows beyond the limits of perception and into the vastness of eternal space. There is only peace in all directions.

Imagine a million miles in front, only peace. Imagine a million miles behind, only peace. Left and right, only peace. Within and without, only peace.

Perhaps inner and outer space have become One: buoyant and at Peace.

Softly chant *Shanti* (Peace) into the vastness of inner space.

Affirmation: 'I let myself breathe in that Peace. I let myself become as light as peace blowing over the surface of my soul. I let myself be that peace.'

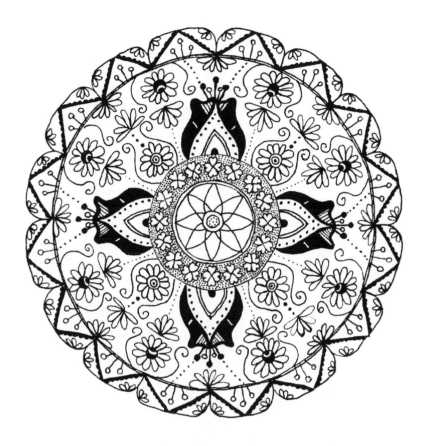

Chapter 3

The Gentle Fragrance of Peace

There is a constant ocean of peace, ever-present beneath any restlessness of body, mind or sprit. How can we quiet the physical and mental agitation to truly experience that peace? That peace eluded me for years. I knew it only as a concept with fleeting tell-tale signs that that peace was real but somehow out of my grasp. The signs of starting to tune into the beautiful fragrance of peace are so fine, so subtle, that these can easily be overlooked.

In this chapter, we are developing our ability to fully relax the physical body, eliminate agitation, and to harmonise to and recognise the subtle fragrance of peace beneath all waves of restlessness. Be prepared to dive more deeply into meditation and be open to realising the relevance of phasing out physical and mental turbulence so that you can discover a finer consciousness of peace within you.

As you read this, is the body sitting quiet and still? Think of all the trillions of nerves cells in the body, constantly thrumming with life force and pinging electrical messages to each other and to the master nerve-body, the brain. Every twitch or shift of the body sets up a jangling in the nerves of the body. Usually in daily life you are so engrossed mindlessly in activity that you don't notice this jangling of the nerves amongst all the other distracting signals from your sight, touch, hearing, taste or smell.

Experiencing quiet in the body requires mastering sitting still, ignoring any message that the body pings to the mind via the brain that you need to move, scratch or open your eyes. Make this the study of today's meditation. Just observe each distracting signal from the body as if you were watching someone else's body. Tell yourself: *I am not the body. I will sit still as long as it takes to allow peace to arrive in my body.* Know that it is a great triumph to overcome an itch or increasing urge to shift your arm. Mastery involves learning to place your attention elsewhere: not in the body part that is demanding your attention so vehemently. Just remove your mind to the brow (centre of will) and exert your willpower by mentally repeating: *I am not this body.*

I promise you, suddenly, a deep quiet will arise from the jumble of nerves that constitute the body. Once these no longer hold your attention, something deeper and more profound can arise in its stead. Experiencing the body awareness as sitting still (or rather body-unawareness, for the secret is in placing your attention deeper than the body) can be as dramatic as the blare of an incessant car alarm in the street, suddenly shutting off bringing instant peace and quiet. We all know the relief in finding that balm of quiet after being exposed to disturbing noise. Imagine now that that 'noise' from the nerves of your body is right now blaring out just above the level of your hearing, unconsciously placing you subtly but constantly on edge. I experienced this acutely when I had Chronic Fatigue Syndrome. Even moving my hand would set up jangling across the web of nerves in my body putting me into a state of alarm.[1]

I learned bit by bit how to lie still, withdraw my mind to the quietening of the breath and to control the focus of the mind. I found that even thinking about moving the body, without actually moving it, would set the web of nerves jangling. This I overcame with patience and determination to overcome a very physical challenge. And you can too.

So, the first goal in eliminating restlessness is mastery of the body. Let's look at what your body is doing as you read this. Are there any unwarranted twitches or shifts going on? Without realising it, often the body is moving. I recall that a bad habit of mine was to wiggle the toes of one foot when I was sitting. I wasn't aware of it most of the time: when I ate, read, knitted or watched TV, the foot was wiggling away. In fact, if I thought about it, I found it vaguely comforting. It gave me feedback from the body so that I knew where I was in space. In reality, what I was doing was sending out a constant agitation along the nerves of the body so that the only calm I experienced was in sleep. This small, seemingly innocuous movement was in reality eroding my sense of calm, keeping me in a constantly agitated state. Other examples might be, drumming fingers, pursing lips, jaw clenching, agitating the whole leg, frowning etc. Take a moment now to close the eyes and watch what the body is doing (remember, the body isn't you, it's just your vehicle for this incarnation and you are learning to drive it more efficiently).

Mentally take note of any unconscious signals and make up your mind to watch the body at various intervals throughout the day to see if there are any more. It can be helpful to ask a friend to say what your tell-tale signs of agitation are. Once these signals are in your radar, then that is the first step in your being able to banish the agitation and uncover the calmness which it was masking.

Yoga involves mastery of the physical body. In order to dive deeper into meditation, the body must be relaxed and not holding onto any muscular tension, beyond the essential stabilisation for an upright spine.

Exercise: Releasing Tension from the Body

Prepare for meditation by tensing and relaxing the body a few times as follows:

Breathe in and tense the body, head to toe. Breathe out and consciously blow all residual tension from the body with the breath.

Repeat again, this time focusing in on the thrumming of energy that is present in the limbs after the exhale.

Repeat one last time, feeling the energy and life force pulling back from the edges of the skin as you exhale.

Take that sense of energy backward into the spine so that you feel energy flowing into the upright shaft of the spine.

Visualise the spine as straight as a broom. The spine is strong and requires no extra effort on your part to remain upright. It is just thrumming with the energy pouring backwards from the

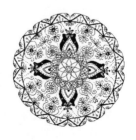

limbs and torso and into the torrent of life force in the centre of the spine, like many little highways of current, flowing into the main highway to the brain.

Exercise: Test for Bodily Relaxation

When you think that you are relaxed, ask a friend to lift one of your hands and to let it go. If you allow this process without intervening by tensing up the arm, then the limb is relaxed.

Try with the other arm.

This exercise may help you to highlight where, if any, you are holding onto attachment to the surface of the body. Try to eliminate all tension.

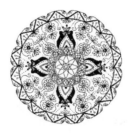

Relaxation involves trust. Trust that your body will be okay if you pour your awareness out of the skin, muscles and nerves, as a torrent to flow into the river of life force in the spine and brain. It is worthwhile assessing at various points during your meditation practice in case you are inadvertently tensing up as your will deepens, diving deeper with the techniques. How relaxed is my body? Am I holding onto any residual tension anywhere? Can I trust and let it go?

It is said that a master can return to calm equilibrium of body and mind in just three breaths. Practise this at any time that you feel that you are tense during the day. Breathe in deeply, tense the whole body and then breathe out, blowing all tension out of the body. Repeat. Finally repeat once more, this time exhaling all tension from the sphere of the mind. Then go about your tasks expressing this calmer frame of mind. Don't wait until later to practise relaxation. It is far more effective to 'catch the moment' to do three focused breaths. With practice, this technique will truly change the moment that you are experiencing.

The second aim is to master the breath. The life force which links us between the physical experience through the senses and the divine experience is expressed through the breath. Take a moment to tune into the breath. How quiet and calm is your breath just now?

Think of it, your breath is constantly being sucked in and blown out of the body by the bellows action of the diaphragm muscle, rib-cage heaving up and down, whether you are conscious of it or not. From your very first breath at birth, this breath has marked the passing of your incarnation and how you have lived it. The breath gives us a very clear indication of the state of mind and emotions at any one time. When you feel safe and relaxed, the breath is slow and gentle, efficiently taking in oxygen and excreting waste toxins. When we feel fear or agitation, we unconsciously tense up, restricting the ease of movement of the diaphragm and the breath becomes short and shallow. In extreme cases, this leads to hyperventilation as an emotional tense-up reaction affects the body's ability to extract oxygen properly from the breath. Even thinking about a traumatic memory or recalling a nightmare can have the same reaction in the body-mind: the body reacts as if the threat is real, tenses up ready as it moves into fight or flight response and the breath becomes laboured.

Take a moment to recall your habitual responses to fear or perceived threat. In particular, note any changes in your breathing pattern. What happens to your breath in a state of alarm? When is the breath functioning easily? And have these any bearing on your emotional state of being?

The breath is the front-line indicator that something is disturbing your inner calm (or rather that you are allowing your inner calm to be ruffled). Noticing your habitual patterns is the first step in actually changing them and taking control.

Swami Niranjanananda Saraswati stated that a yogi measures the span of life not by the number of years but by the number of breaths. Quick, laboured or shallow breathing contributes to the ageing process. Learning to control the breath is a key factor in constantly renewing the body with fresh oxygen, but more importantly, rejuvenating it with a fresh influx of *prana* or life force.

Yoga practice furnishes us with many effective breath techniques to master the breath which is vital to rising above physical limitation and reconnecting with our divine heritage in spirit. I'd like to introduce you to two important techniques using the breath: *Viloma Pranayama* (reverse breath); and the *So Ham* technique, which marries Watching the Breath with a Sanskrit mantra.

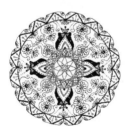

Viloma breath is an instrumental breathing technique to practise as it develops ability to lengthen the actual inhale or exhale and to begin to feel subtle *prana* energies that are masked behind the physical mechanics of breathing. Viloma means 'against the natural flow of the breath'.

Pranayama: Viloma Breath to Lengthen the Inhale

Take a deep, full breath in through the nostrils. This should be silent. Exhale through the nose with a long, controlled breath. Repeat for three breaths.

Let the breath return to normal for a few breaths. Repeat three full inhales and exhales. Observe if the breath is smoother or longer on the second round.

Let the breathing return to its usual pattern. Continue to breathe another few rounds of three full breaths with focused awareness of each inhalation and exhalation.

Begin the next inhalation with a series of 'cuts' or pauses in the breath: inhale-pause, inhale-pause, inhale-pause etc. until the lungs are full. Fully exhale smoothly with a slow, controlled breath until the lungs are totally empty. Repeat for 12 breaths.

Let the body resume its normal rhythm of breathing. Notice the quality of the breath: is the inhale smoother? Is the exhale longer? Are there any subtle shifts in how you are experiencing the breath? With practice, this technique will start to reveal vibrating energy or *prana* (life force) as the building block beneath the physical breath.

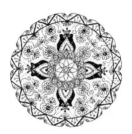

The *So Ham* mantra was mentioned in the introduction as a key technique within your daily *sadhana* (meditation practice), but I will expand further here. The Sanskrit mantra *So Ham* translates as *I am He* or *I am That,* meaning I am the Divine Oneness or I am God. Sanskrit is a very pure and reputedly the oldest language on Earth, impregnated with seed (*beja*) sounds. When Sanskrit is chanted or mentally recited, it elevates the consciousness to higher and higher levels of awareness. *So Ham* is a blessed tool to tune you into the feeling of peace, which is the forerunner of the actual communion with God. It is a very powerful strengthener of soul force and dissolver of ego's chains when used as a meditation. Swami Adi Shankara, who founded the ancient swami order (debatably between the first century BCE and the seventh century CE), stated that meditating on the *So Ham* mantra alone could lead to liberation.

Pronouncing of beja mantras should be as precise as possible. In the *So Ham* mantra, 'So' is pronounced as in 'sew' and 'Ham' rhymes with 'ram'. While *So Ham* is not a technically difficult breath and mantra practice, it is truly transformative. With this mantra, you build mastery of the physical body, mastery of the breath and are affirming again and again, as a super-conscious affirmation, what you are. You, the soul, already knows that you are not this limited form but when the ego consciousness holds court, it overrides soul consciousness. The usurping by the ego of the soul's righteous place as ruler of the bodily kingdom can only perpetuate so long. In time, we become tired of the ego's tricks and choose to turn within and to awaken to our true state of blissful soul consciousness. The *So Ham* mantra effectively creates a beeline for the consciousness out of the mire of reactions and untruths, so that mental focus, the vibration of seed sound in the ether and will to realise the Self, anchors the consciousness in God. I am He. I am That. Each new repetition of the mantra is like a fresh stone pelted on the Sea of Eternity to awaken to your true consciousness of Oneness in perpetual bliss.

The *So Ham* mantra is a *kriya* (cleansing) practice and is a powerful liberating technique. The mental repetition of the Sanskrit words, *So Ham*, acts at a super-conscious level to remind you of your true state of being, untouchable by the deceptive charms and miseries of the physical experience. *So Ham* empowers the soul and willpower to reclaim mastery over the ego. In so doing, the *So Ham* practice resonates to cleanse karma, that is stored as seed tendencies (*samskaras*) within the astral body which is transferred with your consciousness from incarnation to incarnation into each subsequent physical form. Karma is the result of our past errors and selfish behaviours, and is exact and precise. We reap the (karmic) rewards for our past actions. Yoga techniques, and in particular *So Ham*, not only help us to rise above creating further karma, they actually burn up the karmic seeds that we have amassed so far.

The *So Ham* mantra can be used both as a meditation in its own right and as a mental mantra as you go about your chores, so that you can develop a seamless practice between sitting in meditation and acting mindfully in the world.

The *So Ham* Mantra

Sit upright with a relaxed but alert body.

Practise 'Watching the Breath' with the objectivity of a scientist. Observe when the inhale starts, the temperature of the inhale and whether it is ragged or not. Resist the urge to count the length of the breath or alter the length in any way. Observe the exhale: the temperature of the exhaled breath, the body parts involved in the process of breathing and whether the body exhales fully or not. Again, resist the urge to interfere in the actual exhale. It is as it is. After a few breaths, observe if the body naturally starts to take a pause before starting the exhale or resuming the inhale. The consciousness is starting to move into a more subtle experience of the breathing process but be cautious that this is observation only, not manipulation or distortion by the ego consciousness. Keep it pure and simple.

Then, as you observe the body breathing in, mentally say *So*. As you observe the body breathing out, mentally say *Ham*. Try to have your awareness more on the mantra than the breath. The breath is merely the initiation of the commencement of *So*, with the inhale, and *Ham*, with the exhale.

After a while, the breath will be secondary to the mental *So Ham* mantra.

Let the syllables resonate within the core of your being. Mentally chant as if your soul were singing it. Continue for 10–30 minutes.

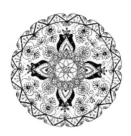

So far in this chapter, we have studied techniques to elevate the consciousness but have said little about the arriving at the experience of peace as a delicate, overwhelmingly beautiful fragrance.

When peace comes knocking on your inner door of silence, a strange phenomenon of a beautiful scent arises. This can be perplexing at first. When I first experienced the heavenly scent of inner peace, I had to open my eyes from meditation to check where it was coming from. Was the candle scented? Or was it the flowers on the altar? Or a hint of the smell of laundry detergent still clinging to my clothing? Ascertaining that it was none of these, I resolutely shut my eyes to distractions and resumed meditation.

I experimented with my experience of the incense-like fragrance: if I gave it a cold-hard-light-of-day focus (ego mind or *manas*), it eluded me; if I relaxed into feeling (*chitta*) and allowed it to flow without hindrance, then it perpetuated.

And so you learn to refine the focus of the mind and give greater weight of consciousness to *chitta* and to override the signals from *manas*. The incense-like musk only deepens as you meditate, bringing in a deeper and deeper sense of peace. Accompanying it is a blissful awakening of the heart: you feel so alive and awake and *in the moment*. You feel in tune with the cosmos. You know in your heart of hearts that this experience is God.

As soon as you attach any shred of awareness to the twittering ramblings of whatever the mind tries to throw up to distract you, the fragrance disappears. The fragrance of peace is so intoxicatingly beautiful that you wouldn't want to miss it. Don't be surprised if it takes quite a few meditation sessions to learn to tune into and maintain the frequency of this subtle fragrance.

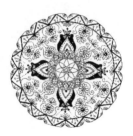

Meditation: Beautiful Fragrance of Inner Peace

Sit upright. Visualise the upright current of life force in the centre of the spine. Shift the weight from the left buttock to the right buttock a few times until you can feel a calmness of consciousness centred in the spine.

Tense and relax a few times. Experience or visualise the rivulets of life force running from the edges of the skin towards the spine as you breathe out.

Practise the *So Ham* mantra (the inhale triggers the mental mantra *So* and the exhale starts the mental mantra *Ham*). Visualise that with each mental mantra and breath that you are taking your mantra is making a beeline of connection with the Divine.

Think of the meaning of the *So Ham* mantra: I am He. Each repetition with the inhale, the exhale and any pauses in the breath bring you closer to God.

A deeper connection is forged with awareness of the mental sound of the mantra and the holding of the focus. There is awareness of you and the line of light directly into the divine through the mantra as a highway of light and of being received by God. The deeper that you go in meditation, the less separation between you and the Divine. With each repetition of *So Ham*, the gulf between you and God lessens and the Divine steps closer.

Be aware of rising through the brow into that highway of light. The highway of light opens out into your inner garden. The brow chakra is the doorway to your inner garden. Imagine walking around in the beauty of your inner garden.

You feel drawn to one particular flower by its beautiful scent like a bee to nectar. Continue to practise the *So Ham* mantra with your flower. Imagine that you are breathing through the flower: *So* with the inhale and *Ham* with the exhale.

Experience the flower like a bee: tasting, smelling the nectar.

Replace the *So Ham* mantra with a quiet but audible humming in the back of the throat. Feel the resonance deep within the body.

Listen quietly within. You are being drawn within the folds of the petals.

Imagine or experience the fragrance of the flower generated by your quiet humming.

Cease humming and pray deeply from your heart: *Divine Spirit. Let me experience you as Peace. May I experience you as the fragrance of peace which flows through my heart. May I experience you as the fragrance of peace which blows through my soul.*

You may be aware of the softest of fragrances arising from the flower as you breathe in and become enveloped with its beautiful scent as you breathe out.

The flower represents your inner perfection of the soul as the fragrance arises from within.

There is only sweetness. There is only goodness.

The petals of the flower open and fall away revealing your inner perfection. You are enveloped in the fragrance of peace.

Perhaps you are drawn to dive even deeper into meditation to find the source of the fragrance.

Perhaps resume a quiet hum, to bring you back to the centre of the flower as a perceived or imagined fragrance that arises from within.

Be like the bee, seeking to find the sweetest nectar.

Follow the fragrance of peace so that in each breath you stay connected and forge a deeper connection within.

Breathe in that real or imagined fragrance and breathe it out upon the world. Be like the humble flower sending its fragrance indiscriminately to one and all. Breathe out the balm of peace as a fragrance.

Learn to use your refining exhale to bring a very fine feeling of peace as a fragrance from the subtle world into the physical world. Imagine that you stand with one foot in each world as a channel of peace: breathing in that fineness of peace and breathing it out as a fragrance of peace.

Perhaps your breath has become so still that the breath is only imagined.

Imagine that the fragrance of peace was filling you up so much that you feel as if you are going to burst to overflowing with peace.

Allow that fragrance of peace to fill behind the eyes as you breathe in and as a gentle vapour as you breathe out.

As you breathe in feel that you are filling with the fragrance of peace and with your exhale you are offering that fragrance of peace to the Divine, as the simplest of offerings.

Making a prayer as St Francis would: *Lord, Make me a channel of your peace. As I stand with one foot in both worlds, channelling your peace upon the earth, letting your peace come as a fragrance, fill the hearts of receptive souls, calming their minds and quietening their bodies with Thy peace.*

Thy fragrance of Divine peace flows to the four corners of the earth.

To the north, as the gentle crystallisations of peace as snow.

To the east, peace blows through the winds of the east and into all hearts.

To the south, filling the warmer climes with the sunlight of thy peace.

And to the west, let the fragrance of peace bring a harmony to all nations.

For I stand in the centre, breathing in that fragrance of peace into each moment that arises and breathing out thy peace upon the waters of the world.

May Thy Peace settle in the earth, the water, the air and the ether.

Imagine the whole earth were encased in the balm of peace that is blowing through you.

Breathe that peace as a comforter to troubled souls.

May all beings be at Peace.

Om Shanti Peace.

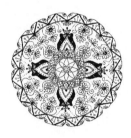

Endnote

1. I referenced my experiences and recovery from Chronic Fatigue Syndrome in my first book, *Living Lightly: A Journey through Chronic Fatigue Syndrome (M.E.)* Ayni Books, 2015. It was this experience of the world stopping and having an inward retreat to discover how to become well which was a catalyst for my spiritual awakening. Every experience, no matter how challenging it may be, is guiding and helping you to awaken to the YOU that you really are.

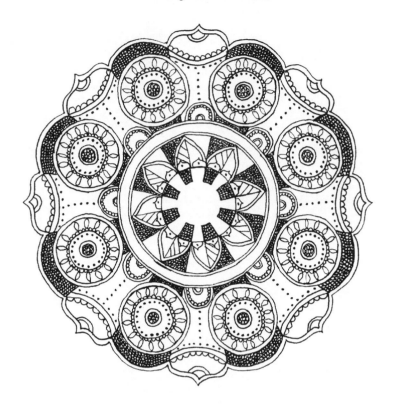

Chapter 4

Open to Receive the Rays of Peace

Beautiful cosmic rays of peace emanate throughout the Oneness and are flowing through you right now. Take a moment to sit quietly and feel the rays of peace. Imagine that you are like a flower in the sunlight basking in those constant blessings of peace. Be open to receive.

Peace exists both within creation (that which is manifest) and beyond creation as omnipresent consciousness. A never-ending ocean of peace exists throughout all eternity as the consciousness of the Divine Father aspect, immanent beyond creation. Peace is also present within creation as a reflection of the Great Spirit.

You have a hidden reservoir of peace in your innermost being, just waiting to be discovered for you is a microcosmic aspect of that Great Oneness. As a soul in incarnation, you experience an aspect of creation which, depending on your frame of consciousness and whether you are open to receive the radiation of peace, may or may not be a peace-filled experience.

In this chapter, we are exploring the karmic trap of desires as a barrier to actual experience of peace, evaluating our current desires and learning to open as a flower to fully receive the bountiful rays of peace.

The man attains peace, who, abandoning all desires, moves about without longing, without the sense of mine and without egoism.
Bhagavad Gita 2:71

As you tune into the rays of peace, we open, expand and blossom. This is a truly beautiful experience that nourishes our soul and lifts us to our true reality. So why are we not always experiencing that peace? Why do we keep choosing restlessness over a peace that never oscillates? The answer to that lies in the storm of desires keeping us forever hankering after something in the material world, whether material possessions, food, sex, fame, power, wealth or a whole host of other notions, and therefore never at peace. Each new desire bores another hole in soul's reservoir of peace. Streams of desires drain away our happiness, contentment, stability and lead, like Alice running after the White Rabbit, to a delirious haze of yet more desires yet never feeling sated when we are rewarded by the fruit of each desire. The ego has an insatiable hunger for yet more things. Each completed desire sets up yet another chain of deflation, a feeling of emptiness, before the ego reaches out into the material world again to fill that lack by hooking into a fresh desire to pour our energies into obtaining. Through meditation, we develop the wise discrimination of the soul to 'see' each small yearning as hollow and charmless, availing nothing but misery in the end. In other words, with the wisdom of the soul, we start to realise amassing material things, people or status etc., has lost its allure. The veil of *maya* (cosmic illusion) and our own personal bubble of delusion (*avidya*) is bursting or at least growing thin. We start to notice a window of clear perception to question before we pursue a desire: do I really want this? Will it bring me happiness?

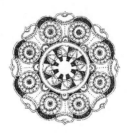

Exercise: Exploring Desire for Material Possessions

Think back to the last item which you acquired. How long had you desired it? What sparked the first seed of desire for it? How much enjoyment did you receive from it? How long did the enjoyment last before you desired the next 'thing'?

Think of something that you are presently yearning for. Is this desire reasonable, achievable or pie-in-the-sky? (Sometimes we may *like* to be wasting our incarnation on desiring inanities or the impossible, and advertising thrives on feeding our stream of desires.) Will it bring me lasting happiness?

Once we open to Peace, it is so blissful that we seek to retain it within our reservoir of peace. That is the goal, so that your mind is not blindly diverted to seeking something more in the external world but stays content within. Our sea of inner peace can then remain unruffled by the restlessness which is born of little desires. With so much change going on in the world, it is important to learn to curb desires so that all the rivers of the soul's joy pour into the ocean of peace and not away.

Exercise: Visualising Rays of Peace

Take a moment to close your eyes and feel that right now.

With infinite love, the Great Spirit is vibrating rays of peace that are running through your physical body into and through each cell bringing harmony to the nucleus of each of the billions upon billions of cells in your body.

Rays of peace are blowing along the nerves of the physical body, bringing coolness and calm. Rays of peace blow through the mind, quietly behind thoughts and easily masked by mental disturbances. Rays of peace flow through the subtle astral body, your body of light, as a balm on the nervous system of the astral body (*nadis and chakras*).

A golden ray of peace continuously flows through the crown of the head, gently vibrating the subtle promise of peace, should you choose to heed its harmonious vibration of calmness.

Rays of peace flow as fine harmonious ideas through your even finer causal body.

Peace flows unhindered by body, breath, mind or thought as glorious rays of light throughout the whole of creation.

Rays of peace are so sweet and subtle that you would miss them if you are focused on the inharmonious distractions of the external world.

Through meditation, we learn to tap into that ever-present experience of peace.

Mastering the body and the breath by yoga breathing techniques leads to a mastery of the mind. Remember the mind is not you. Just as you are not the physical body or the breath,

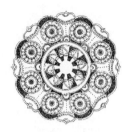

neither are you the mind. It is just a tool. The very-limited ego-focused mind cannot encompass anything greater than itself. The ego is the false self and it seeks to present you with interesting desire or disturbing thought distractions in order for it to exist. When you learn to control the mind through yoga breathing and concentration of willpower, the ego and the mind sit quiet. When the mind quietens, a deep calm is uncovered. Such a treasure of peacefulness just beneath the frenzy of ego-presented desires and thoughts! If only the ego would stop being so disturbing in meditation with so much random nonsense!

So, how to quieten the mind? The first trick is to keep re-affirming mentally: 'I am not this body. I am not this mind.' This affirmation gives your soul or higher aspect the willpower to quieten the ego's stimulus, and in this higher state of consciousness you may observe glimpses of peacefulness arriving as a calmness. These are very subtle at first and can easily be overlooked. Look for any small quietening of the breath or body. Perhaps, there may be a fraction of a pause between the breaths where you can glimpse a quietness, like a stillness coming over a body of water as rippling of the surface ceases. Watch for subtle signs of a calmness in the belly, quietness behind the eyes, spaciousness within the skull, openness in the heart. At the beginning this will be marked by the ceasing of an internal agitation, rather than the presence of peace. But this is a process, where, over a period of time, you learn to not disturb the approaching peace-filled state by over-excitation because something is happening. Aim to dive a little deeper in your meditation each time you sit. Let these subtle way-markers of deepening peace be the trail of breadcrumbs by the Divine Spirit, leading you step-by-step to soul awakening.

I know that whenever I became excited there was a change in experience within my meditation, the subtle shift which had just glimmered into my perception retreated out of my awareness again. I quickly learned that this excitableness was counterproductive to the depth of soul consciousness which can be attained in meditation. With each successive meditation I learned to not stumble over a 'pitfall' of excitableness as each successive way-marker was reached in my daily practice, such as tingling of the limbs as *prana* was withdrawn back into the spinal current. I learned to breathe evenly, hold the mind steady and resume focus of meditation on what was waiting to be revealed behind that occurrence. Trying to grasp at that elusive experience of lightness, peace, beauty, love or wisdom, sets up excitableness in the heart-feeling (*chitta*), chases it away. You learn to re-group, quieten the mind and focus on the breath again, and to allow it to revisit you. 'Graspingness' is the ego consciousness stepping in to wrest back control. Be wise to its ploys. When the ego steps in, Peace steps out.

If you have an expectation of new experiences in meditation, then you will not get far. Hold the ultimate goal in your mind, which is Divine Communion. Any trinkets and shiny bauble experiences in meditation of bright colours or visions should not be mistaken for the end result in meditation. Keep it in your mind that your goal is actual divine awakening and not to accept anything less. Holding an expectation of a desired result is a limitation. Why be satisfied with a tiny thimble of peace when your divine heritage is the entire ocean? It is far better to develop dispassion to whatever arises in meditation, neither distracting thoughts nor feelings nor expectation of a psychic experience.

Some students had some mediumistic training and were seeking to deepen this via meditation. If your aim is to communicate with the deceased, this acts as a limit to your soul awakening. Dearly departed souls inhabit one of the levels of the astral world and while it is possible to develop mental communication, why limit your capacity to only obtaining this parlour trick when, as a microcosmic soul reflection of the Great Macrocosmic Oneness, your true state of being is unlimited. For the victorious meditator, all manner of latent gifts will be reawakened as we dive deeper into meditation. One should not confuse astral gifts with the goal of life. It's like seeing only one star in the sky and being blind to the countless trillions of stars and number of galaxies and realms of being that there are. Creation is beyond measure and so are you.

In tuning into peace as incandescent rays flowing through you at all times there can be a distraction of allowing your attention to fall into a calm, unfocused drowsiness. This is counterproductive. The beginner often gets misled into thinking that this is meditation. It's not. It's merely relaxation, which has its uses but if your goal is soul awakening to your purpose in this incarnation and claiming your divine heritage, then, falling asleep on the job won't get you there.

Staying present as an observer in the Watching the Breath exercise is an excellent way to begin to withdraw consciousness from the body into a more subtle stream of awareness. You can release belief that you are the body. The breath simply arrives. And neither is that breath you. How do you know that? For you, the observer, exists outside (or perhaps this is experienced as deep within) the body or its breath.

I exist therefore I am.

Exercise: Watching the Breath (part 2)

To begin, let the body be rested but alert with an upright spine. Give your body the instruction to be alert and awake.

Now let us focus on the breath. Notice the quality of the breath: is it slow and steady or rapid? Is it cool and soft or hot and heavy? Is the breath arriving into the lower ribs? Belly? Side ribs? Back ribs?

Try to follow one breath in its journey from the nostrils to the back of the throat and into the sensitive membranes of the lungs. Visualise oxygen crossing the membranes and into the newly invigorated blood supply. Watch the exhale softly retire from the lungs, throat and nostrils.

Perhaps you are aware of a lightness in the body. Each breath can bring a lightening of the heaviness of physical denseness. Watch for this with an alert mind. Something beautiful is about to happen and you wouldn't want to blink and miss it.

Bring awareness to the quiet inflowing breath and the soft exhale. Try to keep the mind focused on observing the breath for the next few minutes so that there is no conscious change in breath, simply an observation of an inhale and an exhale.

Is the inhale warmer or cooler than the exhale?

Is the breath flowing smoothly into the body or is it ragged?

Does your attention stay with the exhale or does it disappear?

Is the inhale or exhale longer or are they the same length?

Are you breathing more into the chest than the abdomen? Are you breathing into the back of the body?

Where else in the body can you feel the expansion of the

inhale: the pelvic floor; the soles of the feet; the scalp; the palms of the hands? Can you feel the inhale behind the eyes and is there a different quality as the body breathes out? Just observe the subtle changes of slight hydraulic pressure that happens in the body with the inhale.

Notice what happens in the physical body as you breathe out: there is a relaxation and an expansion, as if you become larger than the covering of skin.

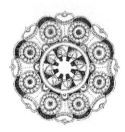

During the process of meditation you strip away all that you are not. Anything that feels 'heavy', reactive or wistfully yearning for something in the material world is not you. You may find that there's an awful lot within that summation but remember that you are evolving and unfolding perfectly with divine guidance every step of the way. When Jesus asked us to pluck out an eye if it offends us, this was not a literal request. He meant it metaphorically: to leave no stone unturned in our path and to leave no weed of desire un-plucked for each stands as a barrier to realisation of the Self. What stands in your way is the ego self, telling you that it's too difficult or distracting you with some thought from the past or desire for the future. So you learn to distinguish through soul perception that which is and is not you. All of your attempts are admirable and a minor personal victory out of *avidya* (personal screen of delusion) on the spiritual path. I congratulate you for each valiant effort, just keep going.

When we become open to receiving peace, it can be a permanently calming background to all of the duties of daily life. Desires lead us astray but through meditation and being receptive to the perpetually inflowing rays of peace, we elevate our consciousness beyond the small, limited, reactive response of ego-centred existence. To have lasting happiness, we learn to maintain this unruffled, even state of mind to all of life's challenges. We are learning as ambassadors of peace to bring that peace to all.

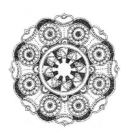

In the following meditation, we turn the spotlight of desire within so that we contain, rather than dissipate, the reservoir of soul peace. Instead of constant little rivulets of peace flowing outward into the physical world, to be lost in the desiccated desert of material consciousness, we reverse that flow and *absorb* all the rivers of desire, thereby keeping the reservoir of peace filled to the brim. We will be charging up the minor chakra at the bridge of the nose and then lifting that focus to the brow chakra (*ajna*).

Meditation: Peace as Rays of Light

Sit in your upright, alert and relaxed posture.

Release all tension in the body: inhale through the nostrils and tense the whole body, exhale and blow away tension through the mouth. Repeat three times.

Prayer: *Divine Father, Divine Mother, saints and masters, fill me with Thy cosmic rays of bountiful peace. Lead me onward, ever inward to develop such depth of meditation that I may find Thy Ocean of peace within. Om Shanti, Peace.*

Imagine that you have roots growing down from the tailbone

and into a golden pool of light in the centre of the earth. Visualise turning on a tap and releasing treacle-like toxins out of the body, mind and emotions. Relinquish holding on to strings of attachment to desires.

See them sinking down into the golden pool of light and being transmuted back into light.

Visualise now that you are drinking up nourishment from the golden pool of light, up through your roots. Golden light fills the legs and lower half of the body, midriff, chest, arms, neck and head.

Golden light flows upward through the whole body and opens the skylight on the crown of the head to connect with a golden ray of light coming from the highest vibration.

Visualise that you are enveloped in a stream of golden light.

Watch the Breath flowing into and out from the body with the calmness of an observer.

Are there any pauses developing between inhales and exhales, exhales and inhales? If so, can you ride the pause, as if surfing a wave, holding the attention without being diverted to a random thought?

Use the pauses in the breath to hold back any intrusion of thought, like parting the Red Sea. You are developing the willpower to create a bubble of calm that the mind cannot throw intrusions into.

Imagine that you are standing on the shore of a vast sea and the waves are lapping around your feet; testing the water directly through your soles and feeling the depth of peace contained therein.

Feel into the vastness of the sea. When your breath has become calm and your consciousness calmed, then you can perceive yourself as part of a Great Ocean of Peace. Drink up that peace through your feet as if by osmosis. This is a quiet of peace that your soul responds to as it brings a peace in the heart.

Allow that peacefulness to enter your physical body, stilling and quietening the nerves, calming the waters within each cell of the body, calming the heart, quelling any emotional upset and floating away all desires that no longer serve your soul development. Realise that you are holding on to those streams of desire and choosing to let them go. The ocean of peace gives you the potential for change. Absorb peace, as if your eyes were floating in a balmy ocean of peace.

Take your attention to the bridge of the nose, to the space between the eyes. Focus the *prana* (energy) of the left eye and the right eye towards this point, without strain, so that both currents of energy converge. Inhale and try to keep the focus of the eyes at this point. Allow the right eye to look towards this point and the left eye to join it. Imagine that at this point a sphere of light becomes charged so that the more your attention is focused on it, the more powerful the sphere becomes.

The eyes are linked to the heart chakra so you may find that your heart becomes warm or starts to open. Keep adjusting the focus so the eyes remain channelled towards this point between the eyes, charging it up. That point may become warm, tingle, throb or another indication of charging with *prana*.

Visualise shifting that charged sphere of *prana* and lift it two finger-widths onto the brow.

Visualise a golden tunnel opening on the brow. Golden light streams towards you, pouring in through your spiritual eye and into the brain.

Golden light, like rays of sunshine, is being absorbed by your heart.

Golden rays of light bring peace within the single eye (brow *chakra*) and peace within the brain, enveloping the body in a stream of golden light.

Keep bringing your attention back to the spiritual eye, absorbing golden light, until you feel that you have a circlet of golden light around the brow.

Commence the *So Ham* mantra, maintaining awareness of

rays of golden light flooding in through the brow *chakra* and the crown of the head.

Just beneath your feet, you are experiencing the ocean of peace. The body breathes in, mental mantra *So* and the body breathes out, mental mantra *Ham*. Just let go on the exhale of all expectation of what may happen in the next moment. Just be in the moment.

Be so filled with peace that the little awareness recedes and you become expanded into the vast ocean of peace. Let go of the mantra practice.

Be open to receive golden rays of light into expansiveness.

Mentally affirm: *I am peace. I float in an ocean of golden peace. I am peace. I float in and am sustained by an ocean of peace.*

Peace runs through my veins and is closer than my own heart. Just beneath the inner door of my being is a vast ocean of peace which is constantly being filled by rays of peace.

Bask in the loving vibration of peace.

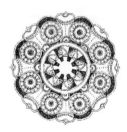

Practise going about your daily life as an ambassador of peace. Pour that peace through your hands, heart, skin, through kind words and gaze compassionately on others through your eyes. Giving peace, begets peace. When you are open to receive peace, you are constantly absorbing a never-ending stream of golden rays which replenish your inner reservoir of peace.

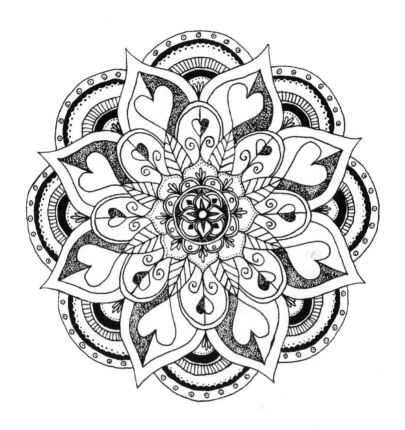

Chapter 5

Peace as a Balm on Restlessness

It can be challenging at times to touch base with any measure of calm in this world of contstant distractions. Peace is the antidote to stress but when worries intrude into our quiet moments as a loud barrage of jangled thoughts, then you become like a little pebble skimming across the surface of life without sampling the real depth of calm beneath. Bombarded by the worries of daily life, you may reflect in quiet moments that life lives you, rather than you living life.

In this chapter, we are learning to be less disturbed by the dream-drama of life, stilling the gross waves of restlessness until we are basking in the balm of peace.

Matter that appears solid is *prana* (life force) and energy condensed into solid, liquid, gas or ether. It is helpful to take a step back and to remember that everything in this dream-drama that seems so solid and tangible is just vibrating energy. If you tense a fist and then relax it you are left with a warmth or fuzziness which is pure energy. What you learn is that the body is just energy and there are layers of subtle vibration behind the screen of the physical body. When you learn to take your awareness back into breath, then behind that there is mind. When you move behind mind deeper still there is discriminative intelligence. Behind pure intelligence there is a still finer vibration of bliss. These are the experiences of moving behind delusion, through the *koshas* (sheaths or veils obscuring the pure awareness of the soul), into successively finer and finer states of consciousness.

The first step is to master the physical body by tuning out the denseness of the physical body and gliding into awareness of the body as pure vibrating energy. Try breathing in, tense the whole body and then exhale fully with an open mouth. Hold the breath briefly and become aware of a warm fuzziness in limbs, belly, torso and head. Repeat another couple of times until you tune into the energy vibrating above and beyond the screen of the physical body.

Withdraw your attention from the external distractions first into warm fuzzy energy and then into the current of consciousness in the spine. Sensations in the body, such as an itch or an ache, may nag in the background. You can learn to tune them out if you tense, relax. Tense, relax. Tense, relax, until you are aware of warm energy, visualising it flowing into the river of the spine. If you find that your attention is being drawn away from the spine, you can disengage it by acknowledging that a part of the body is attempting to 'hook' your attention;

imagine that you are unhooking the thought tendril and withdraw it. You can learn to place your attention where you will it to be. Mastering the body for meditation we learn not to be sidetracked by any sensation arising.

Master the body first. Whatever you place your attention on has an increased focus in your awareness but you can learn to disengage your attention at will.

Being able to master the will comes into its own when you are experiencing emotional worry or stress. You will notice that one of the first signs of stress is that the body tenses up. That tension restricts the breathing from its normal, easy flow into a shallow inefficient breath. It is useful to note: what are your personal physical indicators of stress? Largely signs of stress go unnoticed but one of the benefits in mastering the body is that symptoms of stress in reaction to your body's unconscious habits are brought quickly to your attention, then you have the tools to deal with it. If there is something positive that can be done there and then, you are well disposed to act decisively. If there is nothing that can be done in that moment, then you can use the tense and release practice to throw that worry out of your consciousness.

Act to change the feeling of fear. Go outside into the fresh air and practise conscious breathing. I default to a series of simple yoga *asana* (posture) and *pranayamas* (breathing techniques) that I've used since I was teenager from Richard Hittleman's *Yoga: Twenty-eight Day Exercise Plan.*

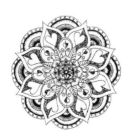

De-stressing Exercises: *Asana* & *Pranayama*

1. Mountain Pose (*Tadanana*)

Stand upright, hands by your side. Breathe out. Take a full breath in, raising the arms overhead. Hold the breath briefly. Exhale slowly, feeling the stretch through the fingertips as you sweep the arms back by your sides. Try to have a long inhale, hold, and a long exhale for a count of 8–15 to your comfort.

Focus on breathing in, not just fresh vitalising air, but pure *prana* or life force. Feel into the poetry of moving your arms in rhythm with the breath. Repeat for 8 breaths.

2. Forward Bend (*Pashcimottanasana*)

Stand upright. Breathe in, sweeping the hands overhead. Bend the knees and come into a deep forward fold as you breathe out, sweeping the arms down left and right of the body.

Place fingertips lightly on the legs or on the floor. 'Pedal' the feet by pushing into the right toes on the floor, rolling the weight down through the footprint and placing the right heel on the floor. Repeat with the left foot.

Keep the tailbone up towards the ceiling and a deep crease at the juncture of thigh and groin. Place one elbow in each hand and swing gently left to right, lengthening out from the hip girdle.

Bend the knees and tuck in the chin as you uncurl the body back to standing.

3. Extended Child's Pose (*Utthita Balasana*)

Come on to all fours. Breathe in and lengthen the spine in a straight line from the tailbone to the crown of the head.

Breathe out, push the palms into the floor and ease the hips back to the heels.

Push into the floor with the tops of the feet and breathe in to come back to all fours. Repeat 3–4 times.

4. Down-head Dog (*Adho Mukha Svanasana*)

Start on all fours. Tuck under the toes.

Breathe out and push hands and toes into the floor to lift the tailbone towards the ceiling.

Pedal alternate feet into the floor, stretching out the heels.

Breathe in to lower to all fours. Repeat 3–4 times.

5. Knees-to-Chest Pose (*Apanasana*)

Lie prone and bring the knees together over the chest, hands on the front of the knees.

Breathe out and squeeze the knees towards the chest.

Breathe into the abdomen, bringing knees to arm's length. Repeat 3–4 times

6. Bridge Pose (*Setu Bandhasana*)

Lie prone. Bend the knees and place the feet flat on the floor near to the hips, arms by the sides.

Raise the hips towards the ceiling by pushing both feet into the floor. At the same time as the hips rise, breathe in and take both arms overhead. Lengthen through the back of the neck.

Breathe out and lower hips and arms at the same time. Repeat 3–4 times.

7. Twist (*Supta Matsyendrasana*)

Lie prone with feet flat on the floor near the hips. Place the arms out at shoulder height, palms up.

Breathe out and lower the knees to the right into a twist, tucking the chin towards the chest. Breathe in to come back to the centre.

Repeat to the left, three times to each side.

8. Knees to Chest Pose (*Apanansa*)

Lie prone and bring the knees together over the chest, hands on the front of the knees. Twist the head loosely to one side and the knees to the other a few times.

Modify these postures as suits your capability and comfort.

I find these exercises helpful in clearing my state of body and mind, aiming to stay present and to breathe in and out fully. It is particularly useful prior to meditation or when you feel you are sinking in a sea of trials. This always grounds me and helps me regain control.

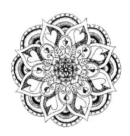

Mastering Even-mindedness

An important tool to master the posture of the physical body is practising even-mindedness. Body posture very quickly determines the mind's state of being. Look to the ground and you are lost in the subconscious mind of daydreams. Hunch the spine or tense up, and the mind responds as if to a threat by thinking fearful thoughts.

Try to remind yourself that worry is just a vibration. You have a choice in any moment: to place your awareness in that negative vibration or to tune into a higher, more positive vibration. Imagine that negatively vibrating thoughts are sending out inaudible discordant notes in the ether to the detriment of your body and mind. You can choose to take a mental step back and resolve to 'play' a more harmonious melody. As a first step, change the body posture and stand upright.

Next, shift the level of the eyes: with the eyes looking out level on the physical world, you are engaging thoughts from the conscious mind in response to what appears to be happening in *maya* (world of illusion) around you. With the eyes looking up, the physical and emotional response is one of open alertness and you have the potential to access the super-conscious state of expanded intuitive consciousness to see beyond the limitations of *maya*.

You can use the willpower and concentration developed in meditation to mentally distance from any problems. Employ your discriminative objectivity to view them from afar. First of all, assess: is there anything that I can practically do in the present moment? If so, overcome any possible prevarication, muster the courage to face the situation head on and act.

And if there's nothing that can be done immediately, take control and imagine that you are wiping the problem off the whiteboard of your mind, just as if you were dusting it off your hands. Expending your time and energy on negative thoughts isn't helpful to you or the situation. Being carried away by negative thought patterns holds body and mind in a state of fear and alarm, where higher order cognitive thinking is restricted back to the primitive brain stem which can only operate in flight or fight mode. Not only would that restrictive functioning of the body make you feel more trapped, it may exacerbate the situation by causing you to react irrationally.

Instead resolve to think positively. Replace negative thoughts with positive affirmations such as *I am calm and thinking clearly*.

Chewing over worries destroys your inner calm and eats up the potential for peace that could be experienced in the present moment. This is when we use the objectivity which is awakened in meditation to help you deal with earthly issues. Once you 'make-up-your-mind' to push worry from your consciousness, you bring willpower into it and then you are no longer helpless. You are strong. Have a break from 'worry consciousness' and decide to not think about the issue for one hour in the morning and evening. Or choose to be mindful of only the present moment, such as being mindful of the process of eating: the texture, colour, flavour of each mouthful. Become so absorbed in the moment that nothing else fills your mind.

An attitude of cheerfulness acts like a laser to negative thoughts. Choose to eradicate worry consciousness with cheerfulness. Even if you are faking cheerfulness, the brain doesn't know that and it starts sending out feel-good endorphins. In a short while, you will find that your cheerfulness is real. And it's infectious! There's nothing like others responding to us with smiles to make us feel good! If in doubt, fake it! It works.

Tense and release is a powerful way to disengage from worries, to withdraw your consciousness as an act of will and to meditate on a solution.

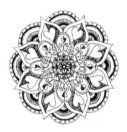

Meditation for Clarity and Insight

Sit upright. Focus on the belly inflating fully as you breathe in and out (it can help to place your palms lightly on the belly until you are sure that you are breathing into the belly and not the chest).

Imagine your breath is filling you with lightness just as if you were a hot air balloon.

With each inhale feel more expansiveness. Each exhale gives you more buoyancy and lightness.

After a few breaths, you are buoyantly and joyously lifted into the air as the earth falls away. From this vantage point you can see to the far horizon in all directions: trees, fields, rivers, mountains and a shining sea. The sky is a vast blue. The higher you lift, the smaller and less important worldly things seem. In the distance, you may see or sense a fresh solution or find that you can let the worry float away.

As you come back to awareness of the body breathing, affirm strongly in your mind, with intensity of feeling: 'I act with courage. I am strong. I am resilient.'

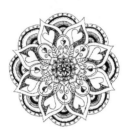

When you have tried everything that's practically possible, just know that there may be some issues that have no resolution. Some dramas may involve another person who is unwilling to change. The lesson that you may be facing is one of acceptance, to accept and endure that which we cannot change. The lesson may be to accept that it is the right of each soul under the Law of Free Will to choose how they operate as the leading role in their own divine drama. You are not responsible for any karmic repercussions that another person accrues. You are only held accountable for your own words, thoughts and actions. That is not to say that we shouldn't offer help or advice, but sometimes that support isn't wanted and wisdom guides us to step back and allow that soul to learn from their own mistakes if necessary. We can always send our love, blessings and prayers for their divine guidance.

Peace is the balm for all ills. You can learn to manufacture the delicious elixir of peace at will during meditation. In small quantities it is the eraser of discomfort and anxieties. In drinking large doses, it becomes the elusive, much sought after Divine intoxicant to bathe in ever-increasing wavelets of bliss. Bliss is a much deeper state than peace. Dipping one's toe into the water of meditation may only bring a mild but ultimately short-lived calmness. Unreservedly throwing one's whole self in will bring deeper, more lasting results. It takes courage to cast off the garment of the body-senses and its attendant attachment to a myriad of fears.

For a very good reason, the Bhagavad Gita (meaning 'Song of the Soul') lists fearlessness as the first and foremost spiritual quality. Fearlessness is the firmament of a strong bedrock on which to build the fortress of your retreat into meditation.[1]

Peace is a quiet strength to sustain you in times of trial. Far from being impractical, your meditation practice (*sadhana*) builds within you a strong fortress of impregnability to the stresses that life brings, you retreat into your inner place of quiet, regroup and return to deal with issues from a quiet, positive solution-focused frame of mind. This is the pivotal point between primitive reactive knee-jerk negative emotional responses to whatever life throws at you and to the building of a strong, resilient positive habit to turn within for comfort, to self-soothe your emotional feathers, attune to a higher realm of consciousness and to receive divine guidance.

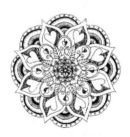

Exercise: Positive Self-Analysis in Your Spiritual Diary

Make a diary over the next month of any ego-reactions to worldly circumstances versus acting from wisdom after the calm and clear thoughts after meditation. Treat each minor victory as a major achievement in the battle to rise victorious over the ego.

Keep your diary entries positive: don't dwell on the times when you got swept away in an emotional reaction. Brush them from your mind as if dusting your shoulders.

Replace a tiny setback with renewed resolve to build forward-looking practical steps in *how* you can establish good habits and not be caught out again.

Write out a positive affirmation on a post-it note or as a prompt on your phone. Recite it mentally 40–100 times a day.

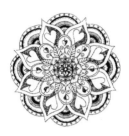

Remember God isn't looking at your mistakes, but He watches how many times you pick yourself up again. That is what matters. Anything that you are facing is not the luck of the draw or being dealt a bad hand in the game of life. Every circumstance that you face is presented in the script of your life and is attracted to you as the result of your past life or present life *karma* (consequences of our past and present actions) and *samskaras* (strong habitual patterns to repeat modes of behaviour again) as divinely directed with the sole intent of awakening you to your Self. Unpleasant experiences are not intended to punish you but to give you fresh opportunity to turn within to seek Divine aid. You've never been abandoned, although at times you may feel that you have been deposited without a guidebook in a foreign environment filled with many dangers to the intrepid soul who seeks to trek to the summit of awakening to who he or she is. That guidebook is innate within you and so is the process of attuning to its wisdom through meditation.

The beginner in meditation will be working very hard in just getting the attention to shift from a restless body and to learn to sit still. As you progress, a stillness develops: that's the first approaching sign of the Divine presence. This stillness opens out into an ocean of peace. Here you have the choice to just paddle at the edges or dive right in. Many meditators halt for many years at that margin, holding on so tightly to all that they had thought that they were and afraid to let go of awareness of where the body is in space, and interest in what's going on around you in the physical world. Remember where you place your attention is where your consciousness is. Each courageous step to dive a little deeper into the ocean of peace brings a fresh challenge to the fear-filled ego-mind. What if something happens? What if I can't come back? These are ego-existential fears of the loss of the body arising from grimly held attachments to the physical body. Let me reassure you: everyone has faced this challenge in meditating but a saint is a sinner who never gave up. I would encourage you to keep on keeping on. Dive as deep in meditation as you have the courage for on a daily basis, and you will find that the rewards are great.

As a ballpark goal, aim to dive deeper each fresh meditation session than the last. Every fresh meditation is likely to present you with recognition of another attachment arising from within. The process of letting go will release you of lots of 'hangers on' to what you naively perceived to be yourself, such an attachment to the body or in holding onto anger, envy, greed, blame or guilt responses to people in your external narrative. Nothing worthwhile is easy. But it gets easier. Once you have mastered the process of letting go, then the principle is always the same, even when you discover attachments that the ego is clinging deeply to. Try to view each attachment as a block in the path to your soul awakening. Also, conversely, each attachment you so dearly hold on to is just a breath away from the release to reveal another beautiful shining aspect of Self hidden under the grime of incarnations.

Make up your mind to experience tranquil thoughts and to discard the garment of worry and the cloak of fear. The following meditation will help to develop your will to deal with life's issues head on and throw anxieties and their attendant attachments out of your consciousness.

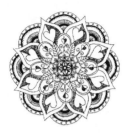

Meditation for Fearlessness

Tense and release the body a few times. Take a long inhale, hold the breath and have a long exhale. Repeat for a few breaths.

Breathe in normally. Explore a pause after the exhale. This pause can be as long or short as you wish and should be comfortable. Try to experience freedom from the clunking mechanics of the breath, if even for one second. Notice that you will have started to move into a more subtle frame of awareness which may be felt as a warmth, coolness or comforting feeling. This underlies the physical experience.

Imagine that you are standing on a beach looking out toward the sea. You are breathing in the coolness of the air with feet planted in the sand.

Your breath flows in gently as a cooling breeze over the brain. This cooling breath soothes the nerves of the physical body as a balm of peace.

Be aware of the breath as calmness and alertness beyond the normal everyday consciousness.

Let that calmness flow down from the brain along the nerves of the physical body. This elixir of peace creates a calmness around the nerves, like the insulating sheath around an electrical wire.

Gaze at the gentle movement of the sea with feet planted on the imaginary sand. Imagine the gentle sensation as if the water were moving through you.

Breathe in calmness across the brain.

Shift your attention to breathing more subtly and breathe calmness over the 'nerves' (*nadis*) of the astral body. These flow upward towards the crown of the head (*sahasrara chakra or astral brain*).

Breathe in the elixir of calmness as it blows over the physical and astral brains.

Take your awareness to the middle of the head, between the brow and the medulla at the back of the head. Breathe in a hint of sweetness from the sea.

Come back to breathing in that elixir of calmness, allowing an experience of peace to arise.

Allow your heart to open with the gentle fragrance of peace as a sweetness.

Perhaps peace brings with it the sound of the creative vibration of God to open the heart. Tune into the frequency of OM by either humming Mmmm... Mmmm... Mmmm or chanting OM... OM... OM.

Each intonation takes you into a deeper experience of calmness, opening into a vast space.

Pray mentally:

Divine Father come to me as pure sound. Fill me with Thy holy word. Om Shanti Peace.

Listen with super-consciousness awareness characterised by great alertness of consciousness. Just keep lifting your consciousness to a higher and higher level of alertness.

Divine Father, Come to me a pure holy sound. Let me see that I am directly sustained by Thy holy word breathing in through the back of my head.

Perceive that you are gazing down a tunnel of light towards the brow. You can travel down this tunnel of blue and gold in a blink of an eye, opening into vastness of eternity.

Look back at your little earthly-self and see all its trials as only transitory.

You exist and are eternal.

In your vastness of consciousness you can ask for a solution to something that you may be facing in earthly life. Hand over that big attaché case of worries to the Divine Presence. The weight of it is no longer with you. Receive the gift of quiet acceptance and calmness.

Come back to awareness of standing on the beach gazing at the sea with the calming breeze of peace blowing through your mind.

Notice how light you feel. Notice the ease of your breathing. In your heart of hearts quietly contain the direct experience of God as calmness, acceptance and peace.

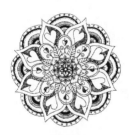

Endnote

1. The twenty-six Divine qualities of a divinely-inclined person as listed in the Bhagavad Gita (16: 1–3) are:

   [F]earlessness, purity of heart, steadfastness in acquiring wisdom and practising yoga, giving selflessly, control of the senses, sacrifice, study of scriptures, self-discipline, straightforwardness, harmlessness, truth, freedom from anger, renunciation, peacefulness, non-slanderousness, compassion towards all beings, lack of greed, gentleness, modesty, freedom from restlessness, vigour, forgiveness, patience, purity, lack of hatred, lack of conceit.

Fully embodying these qualities is both a benchmark of achievement on the spiritual path and milestones of your deepening progress. The Divine qualities are further expanded in my previous book *Divine Meditations: 26 Spiritual Qualities of the Bhagavad Gita* (Mantra Books, 2019).

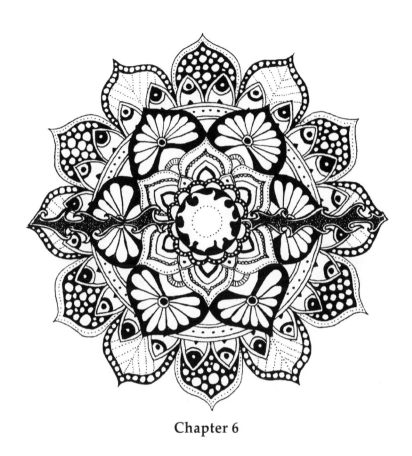

Chapter 6

Peace Burns through Ego Attachments

As your meditation practice deepens with perseverance and daily practise, a more tangible feeling of peace comes into your inner awareness. Forgetting all that has gone before and any expectation of what may or may not occur in your practice, if you have the courage to forge ahead into new uncharted territory, a new level of peace arises from within. Once you reach a tangible, discernible experience of peace, you will have voyaged deep within, revealing a higher state of consciousness giving you fresh a perspective on what is real (soul consciousness) and what is unreal (ego consciousness).

In this chapter we are working with a practice of peace to gain insight into the knot of ego faults (*doshas* or *arishadvargas*) which it has woven, lifetime upon lifetime, and which stand in the way of awakening to the true awareness of the soul. In order to 'see' with the clarity of soul consciousness that which holds us back, let us start with a breath practice and meditation to illuminate our life path.

Meditation: Illuminating Your Soul Path

Sitting comfortably, upright and alert, shift your weight between the left and right buttocks in increasingly small movements until you feel you have centred your consciousness in the spine.

Be aware of a strong foundation at the base of the spine. Visualise the spine as a column of light, like the shaft of an elevator. Consciously let your awareness rise in this elevator shaft through the spine, passing the sacrum, navel, heart, throat, middle of the head to the crown of the head. Light continuously flows down from higher realms through the crown chakra into the physical and subtle spines and shines into each chakra. Visualise the streamers of light flowing out continuously from the chakras, into every cell of the physical body.

Become aware of the body softly breathing. Forget awareness of the wider physical body. Realise that you are breathing in that subtle light and each out-breath tunes into a soft, inner expansiveness. Let your awareness stay with a long, soft inhale and an even longer exhale diving deeper and deeper into inner quiet.

Stay with the breath and mentally affirm: *I breathe quiet into my inner being and bring calm to my soul.*

Let each fresh repetition of this affirmation withdraw your consciousness further into stillness.

This practice may take 10–20 minutes and then you are ready to continue.

Reflect on the list of attachments (below) without inner

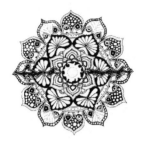

judgement, retaining your calm internalised perception. Notice from your higher state of consciousness, the tangle of attachments which are rooted behind each of the six faults (*doshas*) of the ego consciousness. Calmly let go of any of the ego's attachments as they are revealed from the perspective as if you were simply watching a movie. Remember that these flaws are not you. They are just a temporary blemish on the perfection of your soul, waiting to be released into the light of your soul perception.

Know that it is the ego which holds on to attachments from the past or expectation for the future. Ultimately all attachments derive from some aspect of fear. That fear is not you.

I suggest that you work with each key question on successive days or over a period of time. It is important not to become drawn into the ego's love of drama for this exercise but to try to remain within the calm objectivity of soul discrimination. It sometimes helps to think of the unfolding drama as someone else's narrative.

Exercise: Introspection on the Ego Faults (*Doshas*)

Prepare by meditating: Illumining Your Life-Path practice (above). Close your eyes once more and choose to view that which stands in the way of deeper peace-filled awareness of perfect Soul Consciousness.

What attachments do I hold on to?

What needs to open to the divine illumination that peace brings?

The six *doshas* (ego's attachments) that may be revealed to your consciousness are anger, greed, jealousy, deceit, lust and/or pride. You can skip to the exercise for each *dosha* or alternatively work through these systematically.

1.Anger (*krodha*)

Anger is attachment to holding on to the perception that you have been wronged or that you have done wrong and that you didn't obtain what you desired: If only they had listened to me, praised me or operated differently, then everything would be okay. If only I had obtained my desire, it would be okay.

Anger all boils down to making a judgement on others or yourself: blaming others or feeling guilty about your own conduct.

Key questions:

Do I react well when my desires are thwarted?

What do I blame others for?

Where do I still hold on to blame for my past actions?

Do I hold onto guilt?

Do I like getting angry? Do I get angry to have power over others?

Do I feel respected only when I have an outburst of anger?

Can I let go of anger?

2.Greed (*lobha*)

Greed is attachment to taking more than I need or taking more than my fair share. If I can stockpile more money, more food or more possessions, then I will be safe. Greed boils down to a belief that you do not have enough and a fear of poverty, hunger or lack of security.

Key questions:

Do I pay too much attention to my likes and dislikes?

Have I ever felt hunger or been poor in this life? Do I hold an attachment to an experience of want in the past which

I am allowing to define my present life?

Am I afraid that I will go hungry?

Do I think about food a lot? Do I desire food even when I've just eaten?

Did I experience a competitive childhood where I had to fight to be acknowledged?

Am I afraid of financial loss?

Am I amassing money in order to control my life and feel powerful?

Do I feel safe?

Can I let go of greed consciousness?

3.Jealousy (*matsayra*)

Jealousy is attachment to lack of contentment with what you have manifested in your life and perceiving that the grass is always greener elsewhere. If only I had the perfect house, the perfect car, the perfect body, etc., then I would be happy.

Key questions:

Am I happy with my possessions? Do they give me pleasure or do I think that I need more?

Do I daydream about acquiring more possessions?

Have I got attachment to achieving status or wealth?

Am I healthy? Do I think that my physical body has imperfections?

Do I think that others have found happiness because they have the perfect...?

Am I content?

Can I let go of envy consciousness?

4.Deceit (*moha*)

Deceit is attachment to sticking with the ego's storyline at all costs and fear that it will be discovered as wrong. If only I keep this heinous act or these dishonest thoughts hidden, all will be well. Sometimes we can discover that the ego is desperately trying to hide its guilty secrets from the soul. The ego doesn't know in its lowly consciousness that the Soul is aware of everything. Through the soul as a microcosmic reflection of God and God as the universal intelligence, our Soul-self knows our innermost thoughts and aspirations: nothing is hidden. The poor ego still holds onto the belief that it can close door after inner door, weave a smokescreen of delusion and hide its filthiest secret from itself. This can be a tricky attachment to 'let out' into the light of day. Perhaps at the beginning you can start by acknowledging that there may be secrets that you are trying to hide from yourself and that you can view these safely from afar.

Confirm that you are safely viewing the unfolding secret from a distance: I am safe in the security of my eternal soul, nothing can harm me.

Key questions:

Do I ever tell untruths? (Do I tell untruths to protect the innocent or to protect me?)

Do I find that I spin stories to manipulate others?

Have I ever prayed intensely to God to set up a contract to hide my thoughts, words or actions? (*If you hide my wrong doing God, then I will do... for you.*)

Do I think that I have done wrong and would be punished if I were found out?

Do I punish myself?

Do I think that I should be punished?

Do I feel safe?

Can I let go of the habit of spinning untruths?

5.Lust (*kama*)

Lust is attachment to seeking self-satisfaction and the compelling desire for sensory gratification through any of the senses. The ego endlessly seeks to satisfy its insatiable desires which invariably result in suffering. Through the eyes, the ego lusts after material objects; through hearing the ego craves words of flattery or sweet music; through the sense of smell the ego entices the sense to lust after intoxicants; through taste the ego lusts after rich foods and beverages which rob him of his health; through physical sensation the ego lusts after sexual gratification and luxurious comfort. Lust, when taken to excess, eventually destroys health, happiness, brain functioning, memory and the ability to think clearly.

Key questions:

Am I attached to desiring material things, such as my friend's possessions, a new car, a new sofa, artwork or things of beauty?

How much time do I devote to feeding my desire for material things (adverts, social media, online searches, reading about it)?

Can I look at a beautiful object and enjoy it without desiring it?

Do I attach pleasure from 'honeyed' words? Do I seek praise?

Do I have an attachment to rich foods? Do I suffer afterwards?

Do I desire alcohol, drugs or stimulants? Do I suffer later?

Do I have an inordinate sexual appetite? Do I seek to sexually 'possess' others with my eyes and thoughts?

Can I practise moderation?

6.Pride (*mada*)

Pride is attachment to personal attributes and status, social status or spiritual status that suppress the soul. Ego thinking says: if I think highly of myself then I will feel powerful and strong. Pride comes from attachment to an inflated ego but we all know that pride comes before a fall. The cards of the ego are stacked against it holding dominion over the Soul forever. The Soul is the true ruler of the bodily kingdom, watching quietly the puffed-up peacock feathers of the ego: it is doomed to failure. In meditation, the soul arises and shows us our true nature as kindness, compassion and purity. These higher vibrational qualities are revealed through a deepening humility: I (the Soul) know nothing.

Key questions:

Am I attached to my bodily attributes or beauty?

Do I attach high importance to my character?

Do I hold my character traits in high esteem and view my habits positively but unwilling to look at the less appealing qualities?

Am I attached to the esteem which I feel my career gives me?

Am I attached to the esteem which I feel that my house, vehicle or possessions give me?

Do I think that I am better than others? (I am better than him/her because I....)

Do I spiritually compare myself to others? (I am a more spiritual person than... because I meditate and have a daily practice.)

Do I have the courage to slough the peacock-cloak of pride and stand naked in the sunlight of spirit?

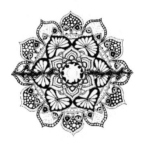

Each attachment of the ego to habitual tendencies acts like a homing beacon to draw a learning experience towards you as an opportunity to realise the folly of the ego's ways and to think, speak and act from the pure, honest simplicity of the soul. Whether you are aware of it or not, you are unconsciously manifesting that experience into your life. For instance, by holding onto attachment to a consciousness of greed whilst eating, you may temporarily be sated. However, by holding onto the belief of 'never enough', you will never feel spiritually full. You can recognise the key signature of greed for food when you are not content to experience the present mouthful but your consciousness is already in the consumption of the next mouthful or the next dish. Through a mindfulness practice we can retrain the consciousness to 'show up' in the taste, texture and smell of only the current mouthful. God is in the food that you eat. God is in the cells of your physical body. God is in your thoughts and consciousness. God is in your present mouthful.

Overcoming attachment to the bad habits of the ego is not a psychological exercise. We cannot overcome the challenge which each attachment presents through the power and scrutiny of the mind. The process of 'letting go' is threefold: first, through the lens of intuitive perception found in meditation, have the courage to face your fears, dirty little secrets too. Second, remind yourself that each attachment is separate from your ever-perfect, unblemished soul, and therefore they are not you. The ego's tendency to weave delusion and confusion and to hold on grimly to attachments is the barrier to soul awakening. Finally, through prayer, 'hand over' each attachment that you uncover in meditation to the Divine Spirit.

Mental, emotional and spiritual even-mindedness is the natural state of the Soul. Restlessness through attachment to outcomes and delusion is the natural state of the ego. Through yoga asana (physical poses), breath control and mind control, we learn to behave as befits our indwelling soul. When I uncover an attachment in the course of my introspection, I mentally lay it aside, go into a deep meditation and then hand it over directly to God or Divine Spirit. I imagine that I am scooping up the tangled threads of attachment in my hands and handing it over as a gift to the light of the Divine. It, as in the attachment, is not you. Anything that limits the power, love and light of the Soul, is not you. God is waiting for you to let go and graciously receives your burden, even a belief in the most shameful sin. With a sincere heart, these are lifted from you. You may see or visualise the karmic threads becoming untangled or being consumed in the burning light of God. All you need to do is to be open to letting go and to appeal sincerely to the Divine for release. Your call is always answered.

Sometimes, releasing an ego aspect may reveal a deep-seated attachment to something else. At times it can be a bit of a mystery tour of backtracking on how the ego has squirreled away fears and attachments from itself in order to feel good. This may be the practice of more than one sitting. I suggest that you be kind and patient with yourself: know that sometimes you can be working on a particularly tangled knot of karma, often as a result of many incarnations. However, with a fervently open heart in prayer to the Divine, God can graciously step down and alleviate the whole knot of karma. Isn't it heartening to know that you will only need to clear 25% of karmic debt? The remaining 75% is lifted off by Divine Spirit (25% through a guru or self-realised master, and 50% as a direct illumination of Grace). So, just keep on keeping on, trying your best and don't be disheartened if at times this seems an uphill struggle. All of the great masters have trodden this path before you and this is your destiny too.

I have seen remarkable changes in my students who have worked wholeheartedly with 'letting go' of the ego's control. Remember, God as your Soul-self is with you, guiding you every step of the way. There is nothing to be afraid of, as to forgive is to be Divine. Each seemingly insignificant ego attachment that you let go of has huge ramifications for your level of contentment and happiness: the effect outweighs the practice hundredfold. You will feel instantly lighter, physically, emotionally, mentally and spiritually as a result.

You may use the *kriya* (cleansing) meditation (below) for all work on refining the self and eliminating attachments as revealed in this chapter. This may be the work of several weeks.

I suggest that you return to this practice as other attachments are revealed in the process of time and practice.

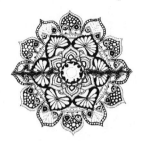

Meditation: Burning Delusion in the Fire of Peace

Sit with an upright spine for meditation.

Prayer: *Divine Father, Fill me with Thy holy fire to sear through all delusion with the flaming sword of Peace. Bless me with Thy loving presence. Om Shanti Amen.*

Inhale. Exhale with a sharp, forced breath through the nostrils, as if trying to breathe a tickly feather away from the end of the nose. This is a very gentle *kappalabhati* breath that activates the diaphragm muscle.[1] Let the next inhale come passively into the body of its own accord. Keep your eyes closed and focus on sensation in the skull as you execute 10 sharp exhales.

For the next round of 10 *kappalabhati* breaths, shift your attention to the lightness pouring into the astral body (your body of light that interpenetrates and surrounds the physical body).

For the third round of 10 *kappalabhati* breaths, focus on a ring of lightness around the head and/or upper chest and on the light that is being generated.

For the final round of 10 *kappalabhati* breaths, focus on a lightness that rises within the throat, chest or heart area.

Let the breath return to its natural rhythm. Feel a sweetness of the inhale and a long, slow exhale. Watch the breath as a fresh opportunity to be present, awake and aware.

Shift to the mental *So Ham* mantra as the body breathes in and out. Let awareness recede from the physical edges of the body to just the soft inhale with the mental mantra *So* and the soft exhale with the mental mantra *Ham*. Keep in your mind the divine meaning of *So Ham* in Sanskrit ('That I am' or 'He I am'). Allow your inner quiet to deepen.

Imagine opening like a flower to receive a continuous stream of divine rays. Let your soft mental *So* on the inhale and soft *Ham* on the exhale, tune in to a deeper quiet.

Visualise peace as a circlet of light around your head.

Continue with the soft *So Ham* mantra as a calm fire of Peace burns within the chest consuming any residual restlessness. Use the pauses in the breath to deepen the experience of Peace.

Stay with the *So Ham* mantra as each breath brings with it a deeper experience of Peace.

Allow the fire of Peace to burn up delusions that have held you back, choosing to let go of knots of karma. As a knot of attachment dissolves you may find that there is another knot behind that one, just stay with the soft *So Ham* mantra and trust the fire of Peace.

Replace your *So Ham* mantra with a mentally repeated affirmation: *The fire of peace burns through my restlessness.*

Finally, let go of your affirmation. Sit within the inner peace that has developed. Know that this experience of Peace is a direct communion with God as the nearest of the near and the dearest of the dear. God is the most loving father, the compassion of the divine mother and the closest friend.

Pray to God in the language of your heart for healing, for support, for you are always receiving God's love which continually flows through you: all that you need to do is be open to receive.

End with a prayer:

Divine Father, fill me with the majesty of thy Peace. Let thy peace flow through my veins and through my many actions. Let the fire of Thy peace burn up all my karmic attachments. Help me to feel a deeper Peace every day; let me know the Peace of Thy presence. Om Shanti, Peace.

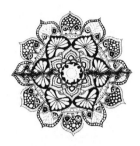

Be aware of lightness in your heart, a lightness flowing outward into the fingers and toes. Come back into awareness of a body that breathes. Stay with the warmth of Peace. Take it into your inner heart, into your precious store of Divine Experiences. You can return to your Divine Store any time that you need to tune into Peace as a dynamic conscious fire that consumes negativity, bringing positivity to the mind and a power to the soul.

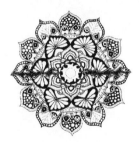

Endnote

1. *Kappalabhati* means 'shining cranuim' and is a *kriya* or purifying practice. It should be performed on an empty stomach. Do not practise if you have heart disease, high blood pressure, stroke, hernia, gastric problems or if you are pregnant. If pain or dizziness is experienced, discontinue and consult a qualified yoga teacher. *Kappalabhati* is not recommended to be practised at night as the resulting alertness is likely to hinder sleep.

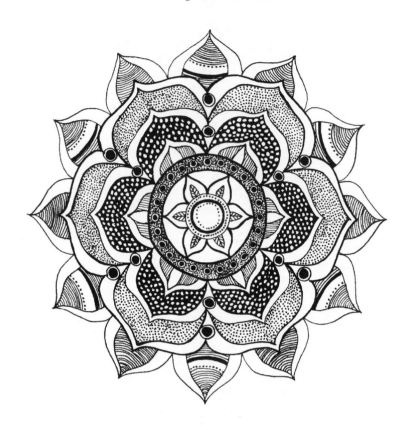

Chapter 7

Expanding into Peace

Peace is always present. If you find that the state of Peace is eluding you it's because some attachment, some distraction, some desire, has swept you out of the natural soul state of Peace. That is, you, the soul, is always at peace. With so many distractions that the ego-self finds more enticing, it's hardly any wonder that at times we feel that we have no peace.

In this chapter, we will be exploring ways to tune into our natural state of Peace, or rather, to tune out the constant bombardment of sensory distractions and desires. If you truly knew the wonder and beauty of living through the consciousness of peace, none of these ego distractions would hold any allure. Their charm, which seems so concrete and so attractive, will be revealed in the sunlight of the soul for what it is: a sham of attractiveness and any fleeting happiness found in attaining it is merely as transient as a firefly in the night. On the spiritual path we learn that what the ego is attracted to ends up leaving a sour taste (suffering) and karma to nullify as a result.

Karma is the law of cause and effect. Every action produces a result which, unfortunately, is appended to our soul until the cause is completely atoned by the appropriate effect, whether immediately or carried over to a future lifetime. Our present circumstances are the direct result of bondage to the effects of our present free will choices of action and our past actions (we are still bound to atone for the karmic consequences even if we have no recollection of what those actions were in a long forgotten incarnation). Although this may seem an insurmountable mountain to compensate for, the good news is that through yoga breathing (*pranayama*), concentration (*dharana* – the practice of concentrating on one thing), meditation (*dhyana* – the state of deep concentration on the divine) and spiritual striving (*svadharma*), we can gradually free ourselves from having to experience the future suffering brought about from our own past thoughts and actions. We need not evolve slowly, nullifying one seed of karma at a time. This is the slow route over which natural evolution in incarnation after incarnation may take millions of lifetimes to awaken to Soul consciousness. Yoga offers us a direct route in a system of conscious breathing practices and step-by-step withdrawal of the consciousness from the grasp of the ego into realisation as the awakened Soul. Through yoga, the soul learns to burn up the stored-up habits and past life tendencies of seed-grooves in the patterning of the brain, just waiting to trip us up by reacting in familiar but unhelpful ways to stimuli in the external world. Much as these prods on our 'buttons' may not seem helpful, in drawing our attention to that which needs to be eliminated from our soul-path, they are giving us a fresh opportunity to overcome a particular seed-groove ego reaction. Remember each moment is a do-over, a fresh start. So right now, you could start to act from conscious choice (the free choice of the soul), and leave behind the reactive habit tendencies (the bound-to-re-enact-old-patterns) of the ego to the pressing of your buttons. This is the frontline of your karmic consequences and each button that you succeed in overcoming gives you the immediate gift of more freedom as a result. Remember, these habit reactions have kept you chained and will keep you chained to perpetual incarnations, until you wake up and take charge. To react from habit means your soul-self has lost that particular skirmish with the ego. Through meditation, you gain the strength of will to disengage, to take a breath to regroup and to reassess if and how you could act. As a route out of knee-jerk reaction of ego consciousness, perhaps you could silently bless those who pressed your jack-in-the-box response and mentally thank them for drawing your attention to another ego blemish hiding the irrepressible eternal light of your soul. Once brought to your awareness, you can then meditate to erase that blemish. Nothing stands in the way of your spiritual growth to your true home in the peace of spirit once you, the soul, take charge.

While in incarnation in the phenomenal world, there are three qualities of karma that can potentially arise from the experience of being bound to reincarnate in a physical body, physical world and one's actions in the world. These are *tamas, rajas* and *sattva*. The densest karma, *tamasic*, is brought about by selfish thoughts, desires and actions which mire the soul further into the blind ignorance of the ego. *Tamas* is characterised by sluggishness, ignorance (of the light of the soul and the higher states of consciousness) and being entrenched in one or more of the six *doshas* (see Chapter 6) anger, greed, envy, deceit, pride and lust.

Sattvic behaviour, at the opposite end of the scale, is characterised by benevolent thoughts, actions, and feelings towards others. While *sattva* may be said to be 'good' behaviour and doing the right thing, it will still incur a lighter weight of karma if those benevolent thoughts, feeling and actions have some selfish benefit. That is, the ego may desire and enjoy the accolades, the approval and good feedback from doing good and this has a karmic result.

In the centre, between these two opposing states of good and 'evil' is the neutral aspect: *rajas*. *Rajas* gives power and energy to either being active in evil or ignorant deeds or being active in good, wholesome actions. *Rajas* is in itself neutral, being neither all good nor all evil. In the battlefield of daily living, *sattva* (good actions guided by the soul) and *tamas* (evil actions controlled by the ego) have a tussle in every moment as to which aspect of nature will gain control over the activating principle. The natural predominance of our good habits is due to a wealth of good karma stored earlier in this incarnation or from previous lives. Sadly, when bad habits come to the fore this is also due to a store of bad karma from the past.

Just by being born into a physical body, we are compelled to act in the world. Even taken to the simplest actions, we are obliged to act to keep the body fed, watered, clean and cared for. We must be mindful of each action, such as breathing, with recognition of He who is the power behind the activation of the breath. We spiritually progress until, finally, we incur no karma when we have eliminated any selfish ego attachment to the action itself or to the fruits of those actions, and act just to please God. The deeper we dive into meditation, by the process of elimination we see with clearer intuitive insight who we are and who we are not. The delusory notion that it is 'I' (the ego) who acts binds us to karma, even for *sattvic* (good) actions. In the highest states of consciousness, we realise that all power, will and volition of body, mind or soul is borrowed from God.

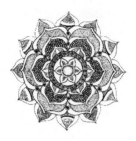

Exercise: Which is 'I'?

Sit quietly and tune into the body softly breathing.

Reflect that the body is not you.

Reflect that the breath is not you.

Think about lifting your arm. The thought, the will and the power to lift the arm, all come from God.

Affirmation: *I am not the body. I am not the breath. I am not the mind. I am not the thought. I am not the will. I am not the action. I am the eternal blissful soul. God is thought, will and power. I am one with God.*

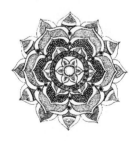

Desire is our greatest enemy. Through ceaselessly wishing for this or that, we are never at peace. Each wistful desire sent with the ego-led thought-feeling that you sent out into the ether may have to wait a very long time to be fulfilled in order for you to have freedom from its karmic result.

Exercise on the Nature of Desire

You may recall the last object that you acquired: when did you first desire it? How long did your enjoyment of it last?

Is there any desire that you presently have? Is it reasonable? Would anyone benefit or suffer as a result of you obtaining it? Is it a purely selfish desire? Why do you want it? Is it possible? Will the fulfilment of this desire bring you lasting happiness?

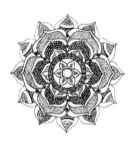

So, how do you go through life without desiring something? As you progress into deeper and deeper states of meditation these reveal such beauty, love, expansiveness and peace that the 'wonders' of the physical realm gradually fall away. I invite you to notice that the thought of desiring something may just be a random thought. But it is when you then allow the heart to hunger after it that it becomes another chain of karma. When you employ the alchemy of thought, will and feeling towards something by employing your free will as a soul, then it has become a desire. Each desire will sit within, latent, until its fulfilment in some future timeline in order to balance the law of karma.

Before you become overwhelmed with the enormity of the karma that you must have accrued through all the masses of desires for people, place, status, objects etc., over this incarnation and all the many previous incarnations, be assured that yoga is giving us technique to nullify a great deal of that weight. Most importantly, yoga gives us a path of action which leads to accruing no further karma.

Meditating to change the state of our consciousness is key. In the normal everyday conscious mind, we are limited in consciousness. Modern psychology and use of affirmations go some way towards changing the habitual actions resulting from 'groove' pathways in the brain through accessing the subconscious mind; but simply using mind and affirmation will not remove the original seed of that tendency which provided the propensity to act in a particular habitual way. The subconscious mind operates at a slightly higher frequency than the conscious mind. However, subliminal thinking and affirmation can only reroute the brain and mind to a more helpful thought channel, thereby masking the habitual tendency. The original seed-karmic tendency still exists, lurking in the background to be addressed in this lifetime or a future one and may still 'pop' up unbidden and bring up the old habitual patterns (you may recognise this recurring pattern even if you have worked with affirmation or cognitive behaviour therapy: the pattern isn't erased).

Through the path and technique of yoga, we gradually lift our state of consciousness to the super-conscious state of the soul and the higher states of consciousness beyond that. Through meditation, we have access to the super-conscious state and karma-cauterising laser of the super-conscious mind which can permanently burn out the latent seed tendencies in the brain. The soul will only let the ego have hold for so long before it reasserts its sole purpose: to become Soul-Conscious of its omnipresence in eternal peace and everlasting joy.

Yoga lifts us to a higher consciousness where we can learn to sit in meditation and go within. We gain mastery of every possible distraction until the ego-self is dissolved into the Great Self, the soul. Like grains of sugar in water, each desire, attachment and seed tendency of the ego is finally dissolved. Employing yoga technique and spiritual striving, the ego loses its borrowed sense of 'self' if there is no attachment, for the ego cannot exist without its binding to the outer or inner world of sensation. On route to realising the mastery of the Self, the soul wins battles on many fronts: physical battles, psychological battles, sociological battles, environmental battles, emotional battles, moral battles and spiritual battles. Bit by bit by continuing your meditation practice, you learn to let go of the distractions that are vying for your attention and see them for what they are: the desperate attempts of the ego to 'exist'.

Each small victory is a huge spiritual accolade, quite outstretching in effect the seemingly insignificant seed tendency that has been overcome.

He attains peace into whom all desires enter as waters enter the ocean, which, filled from all sides, remains unmoved; but not the man who is full of desires.
Bhagavad Gita 2:70

A multitude of little desires act like little holes bored into the reservoir of our consciousness and, as a result, we have no peace within. Ego-led desires keep us constantly off balance, swept along in a tide of hungering after this or that but never having achieved that which you truly search for at a deep level: perfect peace in God-consciousness. Until, that is, we learn to be unchanged and calm no matter how alluring the distractions may seem. Like the children's game of Statues, you learn to remain unmoved and unwavering no matter how your friends pulled faces to try to make you move or laugh. To win you learned to find a place of calm within, beyond what might be happening on the exterior. Similarly, for the journey of the soul, we learn to remain unchanged and unmoved in all circumstances, despite the increasingly subtle attempts by the ego to be 'moved'. Through meditation you learn to chart within and to shut the doors to the sensory, mental and emotional distractions, one by one.

It is worthy of note that it is beneficial for the aspiring yogi (or yogini) to not subject themself too much to obvious distractions, such as social media, fractious people, idle gossip, magazine or TV adverts, but to limit exposure to them. Those that already overcome restlessness, can maintain their calm inward focus and be undisturbed in the face of these distractions. But until then, it is wise to avoid stimuli that results in the leaking or dissipation of your *prana* (life force), leaving you devoid of calm. At some point in your spiritual progress, the appeal of 'empty' distractions will naturally fall away and you will find that you are just no longer interested in the company of certain groups or the unhealthy habits that you had before. As a starting point, it helps to be mindful of what your common distractions are, when and where these distractions occur and to avoid exposure to them if possible. You might see that all the little desires create a restlessness that drains out the life force until there seems no energy left. Through meditation, we can consciously generate a greater energy field charged with *prana* (life force) which expands our field of consciousness.

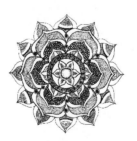

In the Meditation on Expansion of Consciousness, we are using the *ujjayi* (victorious) breath to eliminate a restless mind and realising the freedom from both the effort involved and the demands of desires into an expanded state of peace everywhere. The more that you focus on *ujjayi,* the more you are generating *prana* (life force). You gain greater concentration and willpower through working with this breath.

Meditation: Expansion of Consciousness

Bring your hands together at the heart as you bring the left side of your energy field to the heart through the left hand and the right side of your energy field to the heart via the right hand.

Shift your weight from left to right until your consciousness is centred in the spine. You can feel that you are in the centre when you perceive a tingling in the spine. Visualise the spine filled with light.

Prayer: *Divine Father, expand our limited horizons to encompass Thy vastness. Teach us to know that we are changeless, eternal and thy vastness is behind all things.*

Practise *Ujjayi* breathing: with the jaw open but lips together, the breath creates a rattling sound in the back of the throat (like a soft snore). Feel the sensation of the rattling vibration of the breath that brings a calm to the base of the brain. Focus on the sound or vibration of a smooth, rasping inhale, a pause between the inhale and exhale, and then the soft, rattling exhale.

Imagine as you inhale, a ball thrown into the air. There is a moment of pause in the breath as the ball hangs in the air before it begins its downward trajectory as you exhale. There is a feeling of timelessness as the ball is suspended in the air at the top of its parabola, this feeling of timelessness is mirrored in the breath in its pause between the inhale and before the body naturally wants to breathe out.

The body breathes in as the ball is thrown lightly into the air. There is a freeze in space time in the pause in the breath as the ball is suspended in the air, before the body breathes out once more and the ball falls lightly once more.

You will notice an increased focus in the pause in the breath where a power builds to become keenly awake and aware.

After your next inhale, let the ball vanish.

Imagine in the pause after the inhale, looking out from the window of the spiritual eye (brow *chakra*).

Imagine looking out upon a mountain scene. You are high in

the mountains and snow has fallen. You are standing beside a pristine lake of frozen ice. This lake represents the lake of your mind.

You don ice skates and skate out over the thick ice, your ice blades carving patterns as you move effortlessly over the surface of the ice.

Find another area of the ice that does not have a pattern, until the whole of the surface of this little lake is filled with intricate patterns left by your blades. Keep creating patterns until you are completely spent of ideas for more patterns.

Step to the side of the lake to review your handiwork. It has taken a lot of mental energy to create all that patterning. Visualise the surface ice melting and re-freezing so that it returns to smooth ice.

Reflect on the many patterns that you operate through in daily life and how tiring it can be.

Allow yourself to be quiet and calm. Just enjoy the pristine environment without needing to create patterns.

Walk away, leaving no footprints in the snow. No patterns. No arising of desire to do this or that.

The pristine air is filled with the sparkling whiteness of *prana* (life force). Absorb that *prana* through the pores of the skin and the breath until you too are sparkling whiteness.

Perhaps become light as a spark of *prana* floating in the air, floating over the mountain.

Let the mountain vista recede and visualise floating in a vast space, as far as you can spread your consciousness in any direction, only calm.

Experiment with just being expanded. Expand above, being open to the vastness. Expand below, left, right, behind and in front into the vastness.

Mentally repeat a mantra: *My peace expands everywhere.*

Feel that you have become nebulous and expanded in all directions. In all that oceanic vastness, there is only peace. Allow any feeling of limitedness to be absorbed into that vastness until there are no limits.

All that is left is Peace.

Try to maintain that peace and lightness of being for as long as you can.

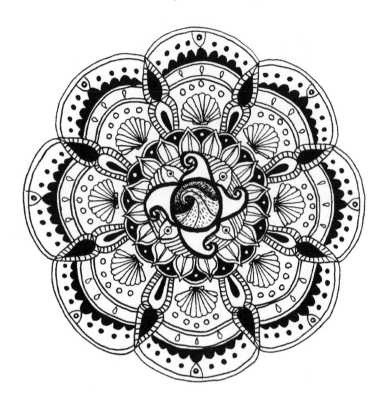

Chapter 8

Ocean of Peace

Peace is always present. It's just that we have forgotten how to tune into that peace. We listen more to the ego's restlessness than the stream of Divine Light and Peace that is always flowing in through the crown of the head. As Jesus said, you just need to be open and receptive to God. How many times do we close ourselves off from that stream of Light through belief in being small, thinking we are limited or closing the heart through mental agitation or not feeling good enough to receive? All we have to do is to open our hearts and receive God's Light, Love and Peace. The focus of this chapter is to unblock your

114

consciousness so that you are open to receive.

If peace were defined as an absence of conflict or war, peace would simply be an empty nothingness between times of conflict. This negative belief couldn't be further from the truth as peace cannot be defined by the absence of anything in creation. Peace exists beyond time, space and relativity. Rather, the ultimate truth is that peace has a presence and power of its own to quietly lift the spirits when the soul has become tired from incarnation to remind it not to take life too seriously. This drama of the game called Life is merely one incarnation in a string of lives: each drama occurred when you played the lead role in the wholehearted attempt to wake-up in Soul Consciousness from the mire of the Great Illusion of creation.

Peace is not merely the absence of agitation or violence. Peace has a definite and dynamic presence. It becomes accessible to us through a dedicated meditation practice and may be experienced in a variety of ways, such as a distinct blissful vibration, a sense of calm, stillness, radiation of rays, or as a sweet musk-like fragrance arising from within.

In this chapter, we are exploring peace as an all-pervading ocean of consciousness. We learn how to tune into that consciousness of peace at will. Peace always exists. However, restlessness of body, mind and spirit obscure that perpetual inner state of peace and it remains hidden from the ego-dominated consciousness. In the moments when you are not experiencing peace, it is because the ego is holding court but if you persevere in trying to free yourself of ego's hold through meditation, you will succeed.

Awakening to our soul reality as God can come with all the heralds of the angelic realm trumpeting the earth-shattering dream, or with the softest and sweetest breaths of a baby that evokes a response of heavenly love. An experience which, for those blissful moments, awakens us from a slumber of eons to another modality, like a long-lost friend hidden in plain sight.

Raising our vibration from earthbound, in awareness of soul-consciousness, we realise that a higher vibration and way of living can be consciously reached here and now. Yoga is the scientific process of attaining God consciousness while in incarnation. Brief flashes of peace serve to remind us that our soul heritage is within grasp should we choose to focus on it. I like to believe that these timely reminders have been heaven sent as a divine aid, often when we need it most.

In the midst of a large crowd or city, the feeling you don't belong can drop from above, leaving you stranded high and dry, sticking out like a sore thumb, painfully exposed within the blend of others. This too, I believe, is a wakeup call: we don't belong here! Our true home is far beyond the realms of vibratory experience of the physical, astral and causal universes, existing in the perpetual ever-new peace and bliss of vibrationless Omnipresent Omniscient God. No matter how many lifetimes you have, this world can never fulfil what you are really seeking. A reunion of the soul with the Divine into Oneness and bliss is indescribably sublime: nothing in the physical or astral can touch that ever-new bliss. Once the soul has tasted soul bliss as a peace within, the baubles and allures of sensual pleasures lose their appeal. Nothing earthly can equate with soul bliss which is our divine heritage.

Paramahansa Yogananda told his followers that they could continue their vices such as drinking and immersion in sexual pleasures, but warned them that he couldn't promise that on the path of yoga the appeal of these pursuits wouldn't fall away by themselves. Once the soul has tasted soul bliss in God, nothing else will do. I used to be quite a rock chick, seeing bands and enjoying dancing to the heavy beat. My final concert was a very polished Eagles tribute band but I had one of those wakeup moments: I felt like an outsider watching the audience entranced by the performance of the 'actors' in their role, themselves asleep to their own role in the drama of incarnation. Once outside the bubble of illusion, there is no way to reconstruct that which I previously found alluring. I thought, 'Ah, this is what Paramahansa Yogananda meant.' One by one each of the pleasures which I sought in this world has paled into insignificance in the realisation of the effervescence of peace and bliss within. You will know what I mean when it happens.

What do think you have outgrown or what has naturally fallen away from your desires? I wouldn't dismiss the simplicity of living with the freshness of a child awake to each new moment. The spiritual path is to awaken to the simplicity within without any attachment to feedback from the senses. Yes, the day can be warm with birds singing sweetly in a park or garden, but the secret is to be un-grasping in your appreciation of these; simply seeing God reflected behind the physical warmth of the sunlight, in the faces of the flowers, shining within the blades of grass and each bird singing as the voice of God, appreciating God in all the guises of creation without trying to capture these revelations of wonder. Simply living in the moment as each revealed joy is experienced in and beyond the physical as it bubbles up from within without containing these. The more you can allow these bliss moments to bubble through unattached and unhindered, the more they arise. Seeking to contain inner bliss puts a cork on your inexhaustible inner wellspring of bubbling peace. More and more you learn to sit within the rising stream of peace bubbles as they effervesce through. There is an inexhaustible supply from the Divine. This is what it truly means to touch God. God has stepped down to rescue you from soul peril after innumerable incarnations to recall you into the arms of bliss: a state of being which you never lost but simply forgot in the infinite number of desire pathways that kept you always looking in the wrong direction.

So, what is the right direction? And how will you know the touch of God?

Meditation is reminding yourself again and again that you

are not the limited body-mind, but that you are the limitless, eternally living soul. Keep reminding yourself throughout the working day that you are infinite spirit and not the ego which is bound by fears, aversions from that which it deemed unpleasant and attractions to earthly pleasures. For you are not small and limited. That is the domain of the ego, the false self. The nature of peace is the essence of the soul. The ego, on the other hand, knows no peace: it is so restlessly searching for this and that that it scurries from one hopeless dream to another without ever looking up from its maze existence.

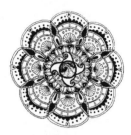

That constant ocean of peace is just a breath away as soon as you learn to lift your consciousness out of the mire of the blind alleys of ego's fruitless searching. Peace, more peace and yet more peace. That's what we are looking for.

The next exercise is to awaken that soul force within your heart, blasting away the cobwebs of delusion to reveal your soul peace within. As a preliminary pranayama (breath practice), we are using Alternate Nostril Breath (*Nadi Shodhanam*) to calm the mind and cleanse the energy pathways (*nadis*) of the astral body of potential blockages.

Pranayama: Alternate Nostril Breath (*Nadi Shodhanam*)
(See Contraindications in Endnote[1])

Place the right thumb just beneath the right side of the bridge of the nose, little finger and ring finger rests lightly just beneath the left side of the bridge of the nose (*nasagra mudra*). (The index finger and middle finger rest lightly on the brow or alternatively, tuck the index finger and middle finger into the palm to alleviate pressure on the brow centre.)

Close the eyes. Through the touch of the fingers, become aware of the resonance and rhythm of the breath through the bridge of the nose.

Close the right nostril and breathe in through the left nostril. Hold the breath briefly on the brow. Close the left nostril and breathe out through the right nostril. Breathe in through the right nostril. Hold the breath on the brow. Close the right nostril and breathe out through the left nostril. This constitutes one round.

Repeat for 12 rounds. Inhale and exhale are equal: long and smooth.

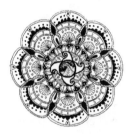

Exercise to Tune into Peace

What if peace is rolling past you in waves right now?

What if peace were just beneath the focus of your body-consciousness?

What if your heart were already full to the brim with peace?

What if all you need to do is tune into that presence of peace, like tuning into a radio station?

Practise 12 rounds of Alternate Nostril Breath (above).

Imagine that you are reclining back in a little boat on a lake, trailing your fingers idly in the cooling waters. It's a perfectly calm sunny day and you are relaxed and happy. Tune into the feeling of the water as it slips softly through your fingers. Build the feeling of relaxed calmness as the water draws all tension from the mind and body.

Visualise the flow of the water as waves of peacefulness, flowing through your fingers. Allow the waves of peacefulness to flow through your spirit. The mind becomes calm. The body is at ease and the waves of peace flow as an undercurrent beneath and through the body.

Magnify the feeling of calmness.

Tune into the presence of a peace that is always present.

Learn to tune into peace at will.

You are not just this limited presence. Bit by bit in meditation,

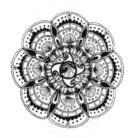

you are learning to erode the ego's hold on the allure of limitation and tune into the vibration of peace which is beneath, behind, within and beyond the consciousness of the body. In the Ocean of Peace Meditation, you learn to tune into peace as an oceanic presence, by affirming what you are, you become aware that you are not just a little body with little rivulets of blood running through its veins. You learn how to dissolve bodily awareness, as if the body were salt, into an expansive ocean of peace.

Meditation: The Ocean of Peace

Prayer: *Oh Great Spirit, guide us to seek Thy sea of peace and dive deep in Thy blissful presence as a boundless ocean of joy. Om Shanti, Peace.*

Sit upright. Become aware the spine as a coloured shaft of light which shifts and moves as the body breathes.

Observe the light in the spine as it moves upwards with the inhale and filters gently downwards with the exhale. All physical tension falls away, like water off a duck's back, as you breathe out.

Focus on light gently rising in the spine on the inhale and settling downwards like a bubbling stream on the exhale.

Perhaps your consciousness reaches the level of the heart, the throat or the head. Maintain the level of consciousness you reach in the spine or in the head.

Practise 12 rounds of Alternate Nostril Breath (*Nadi Shodhanam*).

Lower the hand and let the breath return to normal. Watch the breath entering the body. Observe any change in the length or smoothness of the inhale and exhale.

Inhale, pause the breath and imagine that you are looking through a window of light on the brow. Maintain your focus on the window as the exhale flows away from the brow. Repeat for 12 breaths.

Introduce the *So Ham* mantra (mentally recite: *So* with the inhale, hold the breath and awareness on the brow, then recite *Ham* with the exhale).

Notice the life force running in little rivulets from the edges of the skin and flowing into the spine. The in-breath pulls those little trickling waters of life force from the edges of the skin, coming into the centre. The out-breath flows away in all directions and into a vast sea.

Imagine that your heart is the very centre of the breath. As you breathe in, draw all those little *prana*-sparks of life force away from the edges of the skin, to the heart. As you breathe out, a wave of consciousness expands away in all directions from the heart: left, right, in front, behind, above and beneath.

Visualise the edges of the skin dissolving so that your consciousness can float expansively in all directions in a vast ocean of peace.

Notice any limiting thoughts which may arise and simply dissolve them with the exhale.

Let go into fullness.

The deep ocean is beneath and in all directions, floating. Expansive.

Affirm: *I am He, Blessed Spirit, I am He. I am infinite happiness, I am He.*

Peace rolls on throughout infinite space as an ocean of peace.

Peace in abundance, and yet more abundance.

Peace within and peace without.

All boundaries dissolve into oceanic peace.

Peace that fills eternity, ever extending.

Just when you think you can glimpse the end, peace expands.

If you change direction, peace is there.

Peace is expansiveness in all directions: there is nowhere that peace is not.

Visualise that rolling Ocean of Peace through all your being.

Feel that oceanic presence of peace above, beneath, left and right, in front and behind, within and without and in the spaces between atoms.

Peace in the spaces between atoms in the physical body: there is only Peace.

Peace like an ocean rolls on throughout all space, inner space, outer space and beyond space. Peace rolls through the *Om* vibration and into the pure presence of peace.

Become aware of the quietness of a breath somewhere in all that space: a quiet inhale and a soft exhale. Notice the breath extends beyond the edges of the body. The physical body is just energy.

Om Shanti Peace.

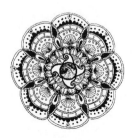

Endnote

1. Alternate Nostril Breath is not suitable for everyone. Contraindications can affect those with breathing disorders such as asthma and those with high blood pressure, nasal obstructions or heart issues. Such persons should not retain the breath after the inhale but just stick with an easily manageable inhale and exhale. If for any reason holding the hand position or restricting air flow is not comfortable, then simply visualise breathing in through one nostril and out through the other alternately.

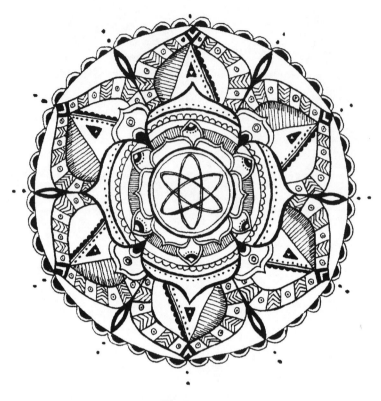

Chapter 9

Peace as a Conscious Vitality

A body that is relaxed and calm invites mental peace.
Paramahansa Yogananda, *Where There Is Light*

Physical tension perpetuates the awareness of the physical body
as solid and is a barrier to going into deeper states of meditation.
In this chapter, we scrutinise the physical body to eliminate any
unwarranted tensions and tune into a vital energy behind the
density of the body. When we eliminate tension, then peace as
a vitality of being can come bubbling up into view from within.

What came first, mental stress and restless thoughts

masquerading as physical tension? Or physical tension stemming from mental tension? Or does tension result from something deeper? In order to eliminate tension, we need to explore the root cause of tension in the physical body, mental stress and spiritual tension.

There are three types of tension: physical, mental and spiritual tension.

Physical Tension

The physical body only appears to be dense and heavy. The perception is influenced by where we place our attention. If we think the body is dense and heavy, we are tuning into the matrix of physical atoms that the body is constructed of and the *maya* (cosmic delusion) that it has weight. Basic laws of physics attest to the fact that so-called solid matter is mostly space, with liquid and gaseous matter appearing to be less dense as they have more space between the atoms. So, if we shift our perception to perceive the body as 99% space with a few atoms vibrating in all that space, then we are starting to tune into the vibratory nature of matter. We start to peel back the layers of delusion that masks what we really are.

Matter has structure in a matrix of 'something' vibrating in the spaces between inter-connected atoms that hold a defined form. That *something* is intelligent *prana* or life force which holds the structure in all created forms. Therefore, it is *prana* intelligence after conception which directs cells to be a blood cell, a heart muscle, a vein, bone, nerves etc. There is intelligent design in the groupings of atoms together for distinct purposes which hold the structure and function of an organism.

So, the perception that the body is heavy is tuning into the belief that the matter is 'solid' but when we place our consciousness into the vibrating space behind the appearance of solidity of the body, we can start to glimpse behind the barrier of the physical body.

Exercise: Feel the Vitality behind Physical Density

Close your eyes. Tense the whole body, holding the energy and vibration of tension. Then let it go, feeling into the tingling vitality that is now in the body. (Use only light tension or just think into any part of the body where there is pain or discomfort.)

Try tensing the right leg by lightly pressing the right foot into the floor. Feel the energy that is being generated in the leg during tension and as you relax, being suffused with a warm tingling.

Notice the difference between the vitality in the right leg compared to the left leg.

Repeat with the left leg.

Visualise a golden light flooding in through the crown of the head and into the abdomen. Lightly tense the abdomen, bringing in healing energy, then relax and feel the warmth and aliveness in that area.

Tense the right arm and hand. Feel the energy being generated throughout the whole arm as you hold the tension. Relax and tune into the vitality which is now coursing through the arm.

Notice how different the left arm feels.

Repeat with the left arm.

Visualise golden light flowing into the head, neck and chest. Create light tension in the neck by pushing the head back against an imaginary wall. This will only be a slight movement. Hold the tension, focus on golden light bringing healing and vitality to the brain and spine. Relax and tune into the warm, tingling, fizziness of vitality.

Repeat with any part of the body that would benefit from special attention and healing.

Sit totally relaxed from head to toe, basking in the warmth of energy and vitality. You are now tuned into the 'something' in the spaces between the atoms of the body. Enjoy the vibration of calmness as delicious waves of energy coursing through and around the body. In time, you will learn to 'drop' the body consciousness at will and transfer your consciousness into the inner bliss of the soul.

This is your key to lifting the veil of attachment to the physical body that obscures your true nature. The physical body is subject to change: it is born, it ages, is subject to disease and suffering and one day it will cease to be. So remember, you are not the body, even as you resume your earthly duties. Only you, the soul, are the changeless 'self' that will always exist and has always existed. True and lasting peace is your essential nature.

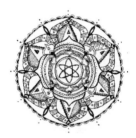

Mental Tension

All mental tension boils down to holding onto fear. This fear could be in the forefront of your conscious awareness, such as an overdue bill or a fear over health, but often these fears are held within the subconscious mind, colouring how we interact with others and how happy or comfortable we feel in any situation.

Nervous and mental tension manifests in the body as recognisable habits of holding physical tension or a nervous agitation of the muscles. Most people who have not 'schooled' their physical signs of mental tension have a recognisable 'tell', for example, a restless leg, facial twitch or restless movement of the eyes and avoidance of eye contact. Sometimes a mode of holding onto worry or unhappiness and the resulting physical symptoms can be so entrenched that we are not consciously aware of it.

Through meditation and the path of yoga, we learn to overcome all fears and to be mentally relaxed and calm (unchangeable) in all circumstances.

Exercise: Observe Your Face in a Mirror

Try catching a glance at your reflection in a mirror. Often our resting expression can give us a glimpse into our inner state of being. Are you holding any tension around the mouth or is the face frowning?

Look deep into your eyes in the reflection. Does this person look happy? What are the eyes telling you?

Talk to your reflection: 'Are you happy?'

Watch for any tell-tale facial reaction.

Ask your reflection: 'What can I do that would help?'

Is it forbearance that is needed to see you through a sticky issue? Acceptance? Forgiveness? Or just plain letting-it-go?

(It is so odd talking to your own reflection in the mirror that this exercise mostly ends in laughter. And laughter instantly lightens any mental tension.)

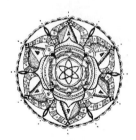

Similar to the physical body, mental tension only appears to be dense and heavy. The key is where you place your attention. With your attention very much focused on the 'issue', thoughts swarm around it, like flies, so inwardly focused that it is a locked-in cycle of negative thoughts. But you can choose to focus elsewhere, leaving the problem to sort itself out for a while. Imagine that your thoughts were as light as air, lifting you higher and higher through the clouds until you are fully in the sunlight of spirit.

Fear is held within the heart: unconsciously we are using

that huge energy-generator field of the heart to perpetuate and amplify a fear. Fear is a limitation. If it were not for that fear, you would be fully aware that you stand basking in the sunlight of spirit. You are always in that light and love, streaming down constantly from God. Except that if you choose fear, you shut out that light. This is often an unconscious choice but we can choose to consciously step away from the fear-consciousness. As a soul stepped down from bliss to inhabit a physical body, we become subject to the stresses of the world. We are straddling two worlds: one is perpetual peace, happiness and unlimited consciousness; the other is delusion, fear and limited consciousness. In our heart, we have the choice to manifest our perception of 'reality' from either realm. The heart is the generating station of our desires; the mystical Wish Fulfilling Tree resides in the heart. So mindful that we as humans straddle both worlds, through our meditation *sadhana* (practice), prayer and will, we can rise up in consciousness, overcoming the limitation of a fear-consciousness. It, the fear, is not you. We learn to embed our state of consciousness that we achieve in meditation into our daily circumstances. We learn to erase old bad habits and mental tension, replacing them with new good habits, we learn to be reflective instead of reactive and, finally, although we still straddle two worlds, we learn to bring through our divine consciousness from the divine realm into earthly living.

Our habitual level of consciousness is found within the spine. In that river of *prana* in the spine, we may be fear-bound within the lower three chakras, or we may rise above that limitation by sincere effort and practice in meditation to sit within the higher levels of consciousness. Imagine each chakra strung like jewels in the spine from red in the base chakra to pure white of the crown chakra. Each chakra has a higher frequency than the one below. Blockages caused by attachment, fear and desire cause our normal state of consciousness, even after meditation, to revert to its habitual level of consciousness in the spine. However, by stalwart keeping-on-keeping-on with our meditation, gradually we overcome each blockage and our normal state of consciousness rests higher and higher in the spine.

Fear is just a feeling in the heart and we can overcome it with willpower and deep breathing. The method is to pull in your willpower and to breathe in and out deeply for three breaths. We learn to use our three breaths wisely, be open-hearted and eliminate all fear. In the throes of fear, you could absent yourself, and do your three big breaths and instantly you have changed your state of consciousness. In the following meditation, we are exploring the habitual level of consciousness and using Alternate Nostril Breath to cleanse fears and blockages, rising into the light and blessing of the Divine Spirit.

Meditation: Raise the Level of Consciousness in the Spine

Sit upright with an awareness of the spine as a flow of light. Shift your weight left to right, backwards and forwards until you are centred in that river of light in the spine. Feel that electrical sensation in the spine from the tailbone to the crown of the head.

Prayer: *Divine Spirit, help me to rise above all obstacles in my life, lift my consciousness into the arms of Thy presence. Help me to realise that I am always held safe in Thy love. Om Shanti Peace.*

Breathe in and out deeply three times, pausing after the exhale.

Visualise all the currents of the body flowing into that river of iridescent light in the spine.

Float your awareness up and down the spine to acclimatise to your habitual 'level' of consciousness.

Imagine that you are in the *ajna* channel of light in the centre of the head from brow to the back of the head. Looking down, you can see the river of light in the spine. Travel forward until your awareness looks out from a disc of light on the brow.

Practise 12 rounds of the Alternate Nostril Breath (*Nadi Shodhanam*) with equal inhale and exhale (see Chapter 8). Imagine that you are breathing up either side of the spine as you inhale and down the other side of the spine as you exhale. Visualise the channel of light in the spine and that the breath is pivoting either side of the spine: inhale up the left, hold awareness in the spine, exhale down the right; inhale up the right side of the spine, hold the breath in the river of the spine, exhale down the left side – one round. The longer and slower the breath, the more it cleanses.

Place the hand in the lap. Mentally continue to breathe in one nostril and out the other, visualising that you are breathing up one side of the spine, up to the crown, and down the other side. Repeat for a few breaths.

Become aware of the iridescent river of light in the spine.

Visualise sitting above the current of light in the spine, in the *ajna* current of light from the brow to the medulla on the back of the head. You can move forward inside the head gazing towards the disc of light on the brow.

Imagine that you are looking out of a window on the brow, gazing through a tunnel of light.

In the blink of an eye, you can travel thousands of miles along this tunnel and out into the vastness of space. Float in the vastness of eternity. For millions of miles in any direction there is only quiet.

Affirm: *I reside in the temple of quiet. I am filled with infinite peace. Peace within and everywhere.*

Imagine that you are standing in the sunlight of Divine Love, receiving those golden blessings through the crown of your head. Hand over any fear into the arms of the Divine Spirit. Fears, like weeds of consciousness, are lifted out of your heart.

Open your heart to receive Divine Light.

Be aware of being in a physical body that gently breathes and, *at the same time*, be aware of receiving the sunlight of God.

Visualise the nerves of the body zinging with the warmth and vitality of Divine Light. Channel this Divine Vitality to flow into any part of the body that requires healing.

Prayer: *Heavenly Father, bless me, bless those that I love, keep them always in Thy presence, in Thy light. Bless me always to do my part with Thy goodness, Thy harmony and Thy love and peace. Om Shanti Peace.*

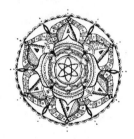

Spiritual Tension

Spiritual tension arises in the daily battle with the ego to do the right thing. The soul in striving to think, speak and act from a higher perspective to do good comes into battle with the ego consciousness. The ego seeks out pleasurable sensations and avoids painful or unpleasant experiences due to attachment to the result of actions. On the spiritual journey, every soul must actively take charge and engage in many daily battles with the sense-driven ego in order to escape the veil of *maya* (illusive creation).

The ego has a vested interest in maintaining an outward focus on the bodily senses and external world for when the soul takes command by going within, the ego's falsity is bit by bit revealed to the soul. Aspects of the ego's hold come to light in meditation and as each 'attachment' is released, the ego is slowly dissolved. This is a daily process of meditation and introspection to 'search-and-destroy' ego's attachment to the outcome of actions. Habitual ways of responding to life due to karma from this or previous lives are incrementally resolved in the revealing spotlight of soul consciousness.

The challenge after each period of meditation is to maintain the resulting inner peace and higher vibration whilst enacting your assigned role in the world, no matter how humble it may be. Soul consciousness, accessed in meditation, has many minor and major skirmishes with the ego. You can recognise the signature of ego consciousness by a feeling of fear(s), anger or limitation which arrives with a characteristic agitated 'gnawing' feeling in the belly or the heart flipping over like a dying fish. The soul, on the other hand, brings a calm sense of wellbeing and expansive openness, acting from love, compassion and kindness.

You may like to remind yourself of this battle throughout the day to assess: am I acting from soul consciousness here or am I letting the ego dictate how I respond? The ego consciousness sits like a little devil on the left shoulder prompting you to selfish or unkind actions: go on, you know you want to. Soul awareness sits like a little angel on the right shoulder quietly encouraging you with the voice of conscience to make the right choice and act from love and kindness. How will you respond?

And, again, at the end of the day, evaluate how well you acted: did I succeed in overriding the baser temptations of the ego or did I succumb to responding with words, thoughts or actions that are beneath me? This daily introspection goes a long way in bringing to your notice unwholesome aspects of habit, intention or *samskara* (delusion) that you can work on eliminating in meditation. Remember that meditation lifts your consciousness to a higher plane where you can rise above and overcome whatever you are faced with on the battle of life. It's helpful to recall that you would not be facing it were it not being attracted towards you by the ego's latent tendencies, and luckily for us, you never have to face all these aspects at once. In the mercy of the divine plan, you are only facing one or two facets, reflected in your physical circumstances of daily life. And you would not be facing difficulty were it not for your best interest to grow as a soul.

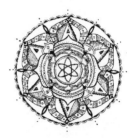

This meditation is to rise above the perception of limitations of body or mind and into the vitality of peace-filled *prana* beyond any appearance of physical density.

Meditation on Peace as Vitality

Sit upright with an alert but relaxed spine.

Tense and sigh out, fully relaxing the body. Feel into the tingling vitality of life force in the limbs, torso and head, beneath the denseness of the body. Apply tension, hold and release, tune into tingling vibration over the whole body.

Prayer: *Oh Great Spirit, come to me as the vitality of peace. Help me to eliminate all restlessness of body, mind and spirit. Help me at will to calm the waves of restlessness and to find Thy peace within. Om Shanti, Peace.*

Take the focus to the breath. Breathe in with the softness of clouds. Breathe out imagining that the breath smoothes over the mirror-surface of a pool of water. Breathe so softly that your breath glides smoothly over the surface of the water without creating ripples, calming the waters of the soul.

Allow the exhale to become longer, travelling further over the surface of the water as a wave of calmness.

Imagine the surface of the water is so still that it reflects the soft, white, fluffy clouds in the blue surface of the water.

Introduce the *So Ham* mantra into this breath over the water.

Mental mantra *So* on the inhale and mental mantra *Ham* on the exhale.

Visualise the pool of water becoming a lake of peace. *So* on the inhale and *Ham* on the exhale.

Breathe smoothly over the entire surface of the water, reflecting the purity of the sky. Feel your consciousness spreading to the edges of the lake. *So* on the inhale and *Ham* on the exhale.

Visualise that you are standing on an island on the lake and that sheet of consciousness is radiating in all directions. The breath flows in all directions, bringing a calmness.

The edges of the lake extend as far as the eye can see. *So* on the inhale, *Ham* on the exhale.

Calmness deepens into an expansive peace. Feel the depth of the water all around as a deep peace. *So* on the inhale and *Ham* on the exhale.

Allow your consciousness to spread into that peace. Forget all limitation and flow into peace.

Continue with the *So Ham* mantra, expanding into a limitless ocean of peace.

Allow your mantra to recede as you experience oneness with peace in any direction. A thousand miles in any direction, there is only peace.

Peace creates insulation around your thoughts so that you can think calm thoughts. Experience sitting within this insulating buffer of peace. Melt into peace.

Let go of any tension held within the mind. Allow your thought-space to be calm and expansive.

Eliminate all restlessness and feel that vitality of calmness.

Affirm: *Peace I am, I am Peace.*

Feel into the power of peace that is behind thoughts. *Peace I am, I am Peace.*

Allow the presence of peace to flow through the body, mind and spirit.

Affirm you are ready to take action in the world with the armour of calmness and the sword of peace.

Imagine the royal cloak of peace placed around your shoulders. With the cloak of peace, the sword of peace and a warrior's armour of peace you are ready to do battle with restlessness.

Peace I am, I am Peace. Realise that you are Peace.

Come back into awareness of the physical body as the warm vitality of peace.

Prayer: *Oh Great Spirit, come to me as Peace. Vitalise my thoughts with peace. Bring Thy sweetness into every action that I do, within my breath as peace, within my words and within my heart as an overflowing ocean of peace. Om, Shanti, Peace.*

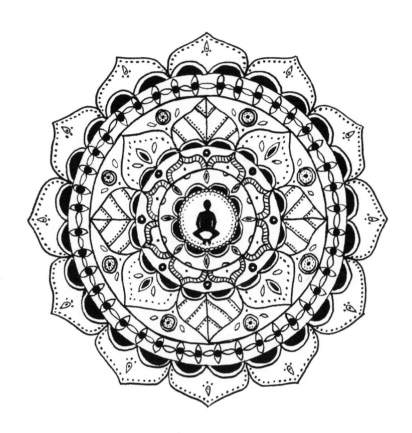

Chapter 10

Encircled by Boundless Peace

The ego consciousness is constantly seeking to divert our attention from moving within by presenting all sorts of sensory feedback or memories of pleasant experiences. So, in essence, the ego looks outward from the centre seeking one indulgence in pleasure after another and is a hindrance to soul awakening. The soul, on the other hand, looks inward to find, with increasing longing, the source of itself, God. The soul perpetually seeks within to dissolve the limitations of incarnation and to flow the microcosmic self once more into the macrocosmic, eternally-loving Ocean of Spirit from whence it came.

This chapter is about developing and exerting your willpower to focus with single-pointed attention. The aim is to develop your soul force by looking towards the telescope of the spiritual eye (*ajna chakra*) thereby finding the never-ending consciousness of eternal peace.

Meditation is the vehicle of awakening to soul consciousness. Once you make up your mind to side with the soul in the battle of life, nothing can stop you. Building up soul strength is achieved through developing the 'muscles' of the soul force through your daily inward battles in meditation. That is why it is important to approach your meditation practice with full awareness of *why* you are meditating.

Aim to dive deeper into the ocean of peace, with each meditation session deeper than the last. You will be faced with all sorts of distractions: chores that need to be done; a phone call to make; a TV show to watch; memories both pleasant and unpleasant, floating up from the ego consciousness in the navel area (*manipura chakra*). Have the soul soldiers of your attention alert to these distractions so that you can let these distractions simply percolate past without diverting your attention from the spiritual eye (*ajna chakra*), the centre of will. Or if you find that your attention has shifted, quickly let go of the errant thought and bring your attention back to the spiritual eye on the brow.

The spiritual eye (or variously named the brow chakra, *ajna*, 'star in the east', third eye) is the centre of will. It is the epicentre of the battle between soul and ego as they both seek to hold dominance over this prize: the will. However, the cards are always stacked against the ego holding perpetual dominance as the ego is not our true state of being and cannot hold sway forever. Although the ego can be a slippery customer, its wiles become, through practice, noticeable for what they are, a ruse, a red herring to throw us off the scent of the beautiful soul fragrance within. So when you sit to meditate, go within forearmed and prepared to let nothing distract you.

The spiritual eye is situated at the culmination of the main channels (*nadis*) of the astral and causal bodies in the spine and brain. *Sushumna*, the main spinal channel of the current of life force is secreted within the physical spine. The aim in meditation is to withdraw life current from the physical body and pour it into the upward channel in the spine. This takes a great deal of practice to master. It is achieved by patiently and repeatedly bringing your consciousness back from the body and its distractions, and plunging it into the river in the spine. This is the perpetual battle between ego and soul force in action. Do not be discouraged when the mind inevitably wanders under ego's command. Simply disengage the lure and place your mind and attention back in the spine, visualising the flow upward to the spiritual eye. (You may have days when there seems to be nothing but a constant disengagement from ego's distractions but know that you are making progress. It can be helpful to chart your daily progress, however small, as a motivator for days when you feel discouraged. Remind yourself that through diligent, faithful practice, you are making progress, even if you cannot see it. One day soon, you will discover a growing quiet, the stillness of peace within.)

Sushumna has four inner concentric channels, each achieved as one goes deeper within during meditation. Within the astral spine there is *sushumna*, within that *vajra* and the finer channel *chitra*. Within the *chitra*, is the super-fine core *brahmanadi* (pathway to God) of the *causal* spine which ascends to infinite spirit.

Either side of the spinal channel are two ancillary pathways, *ida* and *pingala*, the male and female *nadis* which commence either side of the base chakra (*muladhara*), spiralling and criss-crossing the spine through each chakra (sacral, navel, heart, throat) before terminating at the spiritual eye on the forehead. *Pingala*, the warming male current, leaves the right side of *muladhara* and ends on the right petal of the brow (*ajna*). Ida, the cooling female current, leaves the left side of *muladhara* and arrives on the left petal of *ajna*. Before the current of life force can fully flow upwards in the spinal channel, *ida* and *pingala* must be balanced. The ego will attempt to divert our will from taking focus within through these successively more subtle channels to arrive at the spiritual eye. In our battery of soul-force techniques, the Alternate Nostril Breath (*Nadi Shodhanam*) is a powerful *pranayama* to balance these two channels (see Chapter 8).

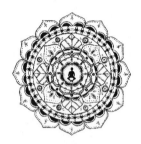

Exercise: Visualising *Ida* and *Pingala Nadis*

Close your eyes and sit with an upright spine.

Bring praying hands together at the heart. Be aware of the warmth of the left hand flowing into the right palm, and the warmth of the right hand flowing into the left palm, like a yin-yang symbol. Allow a balancing of life force in the centre.

Picture the *pingala* and *ida nadis* either side of the shaft of light that is the subtle spine, criss-crossing at the main chakras.

Observe the *pingala* channel: right of base chakra, flowing up into the sacral chakra. Exiting left of the sacral chakra, *pingala* flows upwards into the left of the navel chakra. *Pingala* exits on the right of the navel chakra and flowing up into the right of the heart chakra. Leaving the left side of the heart chakra, *pingala* enters the left side of the throat chakra. Leaving right of the throat, it arrives on the right side of the brow.

Observe the *ida* channel: left of base chakra, flowing up

into the sacral chakra. Exiting the right of the sacral chakra, *ida* spirals upwards into the right of the navel chakra. Leaving left of the navel, *ida* flows up into the left of the heart chakra. Leaving the right side of the heart chakra, *ida* enters the right side of the throat chakra. Leaving left of the throat, it terminates on the left side of the brow.

Visualise the brow chakra (Spiritual eye) between and slightly above the two physical eyes as the termination of *ida, pingala* and spinal channels.

Visualise the two petals of the brow chakra as where rivers of *ida* and *pingala* empty into the power of the spiritual eye.

Imagine that you are looking through the spiritual eye as an aperture of light in the centre.

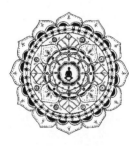

Exercise: Visualising the Anatomy of the Subtle Spine

Close your eyes and sit with an upright spine.

Rest the hands on the thighs. Touch the tips of the right fore-finger and right thumb together. Touch left fore-finger and left thumb together in the *jnanna mudra*. Concentrate on the flow of life force through the connected finger and thumb. There may be a warmth flowing up the arms and emptying behind the heart. Stay with *jnanna mudra* until there is a sense of withdrawal from the edges of the body and into the centre.

Allow the hands to relax and be aware of the body breathing gently.

Visualise the spine as a hollow shaft of light. Within the physical spine, and superimposed upon it, are the subtle astral spine and the super-fine *causal* spine.

Sink back from being forward-focused and into the river of consciousness in the spine.

Visualise the physical spine as lumps of bone, stacked one upon the other and in the centre the spinal nerve pathway flowing upward into the great neural network of the brain.

Picture the astral spine in a horizontal sectional view as a column of light surrounded by two concentric circles. The outermost covering is *sushumna*, the sheath of the astral spine.

Picture moving within to an even finer state of consciousness (*vajna*) within *sushumna*. Within the centre of *vajna* there is an even finer channel called *chitra*.

Visualise the super-fine causal spine superimposed as a fine vibration within the astral spine, termed *bramha nadi* (pathway to God).

Feel into the current of life force in all three spines flowing upwards into the skull.

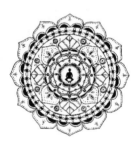

In gaining mastery of the centre of will, the direction that the physical eyes are facing, even behind closed eyes, is highly important in directing the current to go within. Where the eyes are 'looking' is where the attention is focused. The electrical *prana* current of the physical eyes must be trained to focus on the single point of the spiritual eye in order to gain command of the will in the battle between the ego and the soul.

Mastering the gaze of the physical eyes is vital in mastering control of the mind. In yoga meditation, we train the eyes to focus towards the *ajna* chakra and to imagine (imagination is the precursor to actually seeing) that we are gazing toward a pulsating disc of light on the brow. The two channels of the physical eyes, one relating to *ida* and the other relating to *pingala*, become single at that point. The key awareness of the meeting of prana-light from the left eye meeting prana-light from the right eye coming to the one point on the brow, is the sensation of pressure, calmness or light, or sometimes all three. The more that you can focus both eyes on the seat of consciousness on the brow, you more you develop your seat of super-conscious will, the *ajna* chakra. This is the will of the soul to move inwards towards God, overriding the ego's desire to dissipate the consciousness outward into the many distractions of the external world through a sense-orientated mind.

In meditation when we learn to refocus the current of the eyes into the single current of the spiritual eye, it exerts a strong pull of life force to withdraw the life currently at the edges of the skin. When this is mastered, it results in the vision expanding from the normal biopic vision of the physical eyes into the spherical vision of the astral body. Although there may be some discomfort at first in bringing the eyes to gaze at the point between and slightly above them on the brow, with practice this will become easier. Hold the gaze steady without allowing the eyes to flicker or move around, you will start to see the spherical eye as a golden halo surrounding electric blue with a five-pointed white star in the centre. It takes a great deal of practice to see the star in the centre, so do not be discouraged if you do not see it straight away.

In respect of other lights and visions which may be seen in the spiritual eye, treat these as distractions on the spiritual path. There is a psychic knot (*rudha granthi*) in *ajna* chakra which is a divinely-placed barrier to progressing on the spiritual path until you are ready. If there is a desire to see psychic phenomena, this is best not to be entertained; seeing psychic phenomena does not indicate true spiritual progress but simply that you have tapped into the innate sight of the astral body. It is not until you are willing to see the One light behind all these astral projections that the spiritual eye will open fully for you. Your will is determined by whatever you desire. Once you make up your mind (that's the key phrase here: once you make up your mind to stay on track for spiritual progress and to see God and only God, for then you are executing your Divine Will as a microcosmic aspect of the Great Macrocosm, and it will manifest) nothing can stop you.

The true mark of spiritual progress is not seeing saints, phenomena or visions but how calmly you are able to endure without restlessness circumstances that arise in the physical world, in the cold, hard light of day.

Meditation practice will consist of maintaining focus fixedly on this point which, when you pour all your consciousness into it, operates a trigger to withdraw life current from the body to flood the spiritual eye with brilliant white light. Although this may change in colour and shape depending on the vibration of your thoughts, white light is very common in the beginning. Once you become firmly established in your focus on the brow, all variations in colours of light settle into the one true spiritual eye as a sphere of shimmering gold with a deep blue centre. Train yourself to look directly towards the centre of the blue. With deep attention, you may catch glimpse of the white star in the centre. It takes a great deal of practice to steady the thought perceptions of the astral eye until you can hold the light steady on the star. The star is the doorway to the higher states of consciousness: Christ Consciousness and Cosmic Consciousness. These must be mastered in order to travel through the star into *kaivalya* (soul liberation) from the bondage of karma and repeated incarnations.

At times the spiritual eye may seem very far away, but the more intensely focused your attention is, without any deviation of attention, the closer or larger the eye becomes. Until it can appear to occupy not only frontal vision as in the physical eyes, but the whole head space so that you can see in all directions (without moving the physical body). In fact, the spiritual eye is beyond space or time as it is not limited to earthly constraints of linear time or seeing in three dimensions.

You will find that one side of the body is naturally steadier in being able to hold the focus on the single point of the brow. You may find that one eye keeps wandering away. This is an indication of an imbalance or blockage in the chakras, especially the navel and the heart. It can be helpful to place the seat of your attention in directing the current of the steadier eye until the will is firmly anchored in the brow chakra, before transferring that calm attention and focus to the other eye. In other words, if there is an imbalance of focus, use the stronger focus of one eye to influence the focus of the weaker eye by bringing it into accord.

The light of the body is the eye: if therefore thine eye be single, thy whole body shall be full of light.
Matthew 6:22–23

Exercise: Train the Physical Eyes towards the Brow
Sit upright and close the eyes.

Observe the passage of the breath in the bridge of the nose: cool air on the inhale and warmer air on the exhale.

Touch the brow centre with one finger (slightly above the eyebrows). Then let the hand rest.

Let the eyes look up towards the feeling of that point, with closed lids.

Try to keep the soft focus of both eyes trained to that point.

If the eyes flicker, keep bringing them under your command.

Have patience while the eye muscles get used to this, at first, unfamiliar position. If there is discomfort, ease back on effort.

Check with your doctor or optician if you are unsure, although this exercise should be perfectly within the range of comfort for most people. It is sometimes helpful to focus on an imaginary point 5 inches in front of the brow.

The main point is that you look up, shifting the gaze from the level of the two eyes, to look out from the level of the brow.

Remember that you are triggering a change in consciousness by making binary vision single. This shift may be experienced in small stages: expansion of consciousness; wandering of focus with the eyes; refocusing the eyes; expansion to a slightly higher frequency of consciousness; wandering of the focus; refocusing the eyes; expansion to an even higher frequency of consciousness etc.

Stay with the steadiness of the eye's gaze. Aim to hold for one second without deviation. Then two seconds. Develop longer and longer periods of focusing the eyes on the single point. When you bring both eye-currents to the same point, there is a sensation of calm. Aim for these moments of calm.

Practise for one minute and extend this a minute a day to twenty minutes.

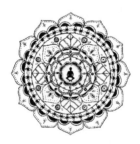

Meditation: Expansiveness of Peace

Prayer: *O Spirit, I Bow to Thee in front of me, behind me, on the left and on the right. I bow to Thee above and beneath me. I bow to thee within and without. O Lord, Thou are omnipresent. Awaken me in Thy Omnipresence. Om Shanti Peace.*

Close the eyelids. Look up under the closed lids to focus the current of attention of the physical eyes at the spiritual eye.

Introduce the mental *So Ham* mantra: *So* on the inhale and *Ham* on the exhale; while maintaining focus and awareness on the spiritual eye. *So* draws a cool calmness that ripples through the brain and the spiritual eye with the inhale. *Ham* brings the sensation of a slight warming current through the brain and the brow with the exhale. Keep bringing left eye and right eye to meet on the brow centre. Maintain the mantra with the focus of the eyes for ten minutes.

Replace the mental mantra with an audible hum. Hum softly, giving full attention to the *mmmm* vibration which vibrates the back of the head creating ripples of sound along the *ajna* channel, from the back of the head arriving at the spiritual eye. Repeat for two or three minutes.

Experience an expansiveness of your boundless omnipresence: behind and in front, above and beneath, left and right, within and without. Your body has become infinity.

There is a halo of peace encircling your body. You are surrounded by peace in all directions and encircled by peace.

Experience gentle waves of peace flowing within and everywhere.

Affirmation: *I am boundless peace. I am expansiveness.*

Allow any perception of limitedness or littleness to simply fall away. Spread your consciousness over infinite space.

In all directions, there is only peace: the vastness of peace. Everywhere at all times there is only peace.

If you take your consciousness a thousand miles in any direction, there is only the boundlessness of infinite peace. You are held in a cradle of peace.

Gently become aware of the softly breathing body and choose to experience the expansiveness of peace.

Experience peace: in the lungs; the four chambers of the physical heart and in the spine.

Visualise the root of the heart chakra in the spine. Visualise its twelve radiating petals, rotating upward in the spine to face the spiritual sun of *sahasrara* (crown chakra). Dissolve any 'littleness' or sense of being 'small' so that the petals of the heart can open expansively.

Breathe into each petal of the heart, allowing it to be clear and open so that the clarity of peace can flow through each one.

Breathe in peace. Breathe out peacefulness into the bubble of light around yourself: peacefulness in front; peacefulness behind, as if lying back on the softness of a feather bed; peace to the left and right expressed through the hands as peace-filled movements; peace below as a gentle connection with the earth so that your feet walk lightly; peace above as a golden aura of light; peace within the body.

Visualise peace as a golden bubble of light around the body. Breathe golden light into the lungs to fortify them with peace so that your breath can be calm and peaceful, expressing calm and peaceful words from a calm and peaceful brain, and calm and peaceful thoughts.

Breathe in more deeply, breathing in peace and breathing out peace. Be conscious of that golden bubble of light as a vibration of peace that expands out across the world. So that wherever you tread, you bring peace, as a peace-maker on the planet.

Think of others across the planet in need of healing prayers. Think of them in peace, bathing in your prayer.

Peace spreads out across the planet. May Peace Prevail on Earth.

Prayer: *Oh Spirit, come to me as peace. Let Thy peace be upon my lips, bringing words of solace. Let Thy peace be upon my hands, doing peaceful works. May Thy peace be upon my heart bringing Thy peacefulness wherever I go. Om, Shanti, Peace, Amen.*

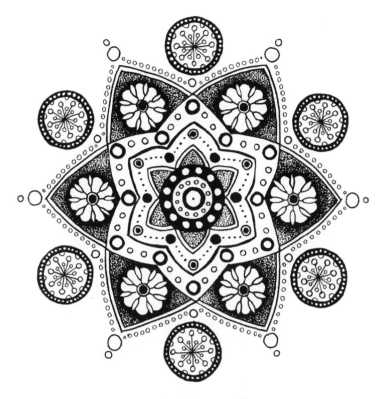

Chapter 11

Peace in Every Pore of My Being

There once lived a famous sculptor in India, famed for his majestic stone elephants, so life-like that they seemed about to trumpet, march off the plinth and join their kin in the jungle. The fame of this sculptor reached the ears of the Maharaja who went to see this skilled craftsman for himself, marvelling at the magnificent exactitude of his sculptures. Standing before the sculptor, the great man asked, *What is the secret of your artistry?*

The sculptor was silent for a time as if dredging up words from a great depth. *When a fresh block of granite sits before me, I look deep within its shape, viewing it from all angles. At first, it is just a lump of stone but as I watch, the faint outline of its inner shape starts to appear to me. Imperceptible as a ghost of an outline, the image becomes clearer and clearer until at last I can see the elephant that is hidden in the block of stone. Then I hold the image of the elephant that the stone wants to be in my head as I chisel. I chip away all that is not the elephant, to reveal the elephant itself.*

This is an allegory for the process of meditation. With the patience of meditation, gradually you chip away all that you are not, to reveal that which you are: the light of the indwelling soul.

It's helpful to keep reminding yourself that you, the soul, are perfect. You have always existed and will always exist, untouchable, changeless and unharmed by illness, sorrows, karma, birth or death. These experiences are just temporary blemishes that obscure the perfection of the soul. Anything that is temporary is not the soul. The physical body is temporary and subject to the changes of birth, ageing, illness and death, therefore you are not the body. The breath is in constant flux and therefore you are not the breath. You existed before this incarnation and therefore are not any of the roles that you play: mother, father, sister, brother, husband, wife, daughter, son, friend, colleague, teacher, student, employee and so on, for you have played many other roles before. To identify with a role in the divine play (*lila*) is to be limited. Chip away all that you are not and you will reveal the god-light of your soul within.

Each meditation session may bring up another aspect that is not you. If there is a strong karmic attachment you may find that you are working to release the ego's grip on the attachment to that 'difference' for several days. You can tell that it is other than the soul because you are observing it as separate from 'you'. It is also recognisable in that the mere thought of letting it go or not operating through that mode may cause emotional pain: that is attachment. Attachment to objects, people, place, status and even this body are all 'separateness'. One need never lose sight of the goal of incarnation which is to realise who you are and to become reunited with the Oneness. A belief in separateness is what keeps you separate from that Great Spirit.

This summed up in my favourite sloka from the Bhagavad Gita.

Fix thy mind on Me, be devoted to Me, resign all things to Me, bow down to Me. Thou shalt attain Me; truly do I promise unto thee, [for] thou art dear to Me.

Bhagavad Gita 18:65

The Divine Lord says: Resign all things to me. Hand them over, the foul and the fair alike within. For there is nothing that is hidden from God, much as you in your naivety may like to hide deeds from yourself which were done in anger or selfishness, these are transparent to God. Bringing everything, warts and all, out into the open before God is most healing.

In order for there to be peace within, there must be no harbouring of resentments or ill will towards anyone or yourself. What I found was that I felt lighter with each release. In meditation, I would use my hands and visualise lifting some weight of karma out of my body (whatever had come to my attention as a 'reaction' to daily events, perhaps angry at what someone said, I knew that I could be in charge of knee-jerk responses if I bring it out into the open before God in prayer, and in doing so wrest that control from the ego), lifting my hands in offering to a loving God. All offerings are accepted.

Cast your burden on the Lord, and He will sustain you (Psalm 55:22).

Karmic seeds of your past actions and thoughts are stored in the astral body from lifetime to lifetime. Depending on where these are stored in the body and how toxic (or evil) these are, they can manifest in the physical body as ailments. For example: lungs hold onto grief and sadness, the kidneys and bladder hold onto fear, stomach holds onto anger. If you are experiencing a physical illness it may be helpful to go within in meditation and ask that part of the body what it is holding onto. You may have no memory of why you develop attachment to a fear or anger from a past life as, mercifully, the divine curtain comes down between incarnations so that we get a fresh chance to do our best without the hindrance of past life memories. However, through meditation, we have the means to go within, to chip away the attachments of the past and to see, with the eyes of the soul, our shining self.

You are a child of God, no lesser for any of your past karma. In the following exercise, an appeal is made to the Divine Mother aspect who loves you unconditionally with the forgiving love of a mother for her beloved child. Remember, God sees your heart and knows that you genuinely are seeking to know yourself. Approach God with your heart open and mind set on letting go of the past and becoming awake, you will always be heard.

Exercise: Releasing Karma

Prayer: *Divine Mother, lifetime after lifetime I have hidden from Thee. No more do I hide. Help me. Make me clean and lift me up in the sunlight of Thy love. Om Shanti Amen*

Become still in meditation.

Visualise or feel the Divine Mother coming close, bestowing Her gentle blessings. Perhaps she is already lifting away your burdens as you open to spirit.

Or perhaps she is revealing the weight which you hold onto as a tightness harboured somewhere in the body. Imagine that you are scooping that weight on your hands and lifting it out of your body. Offer it to Divine Mother as if you were offering the highest and best of yourself. Keep offering holding the space and silently praying to Divine Mother. You may feel, see or imagine that something is lifted out of you.

Visualise or feel a great light shining upon you as you receive the healing blessings of the Divine Mother in white or golden light.

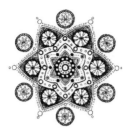

Sometimes, this exercise may have to go deeper. If I found a pang of not-wanting-to-let-go within me, I used the incisive knife of my will to 'unhook' the barb of my attachment to a deep feeling beneath the initial burden. Try to sum up the feeling in one word, as separate from the storyline around it. It could be blame, judgement, resentment, anger, guilt, pride, envy, fear of loss, hate or sadness, to name but a few. Imagine prising up that root of attachment under the loving guidance of Divine Mother and lifting it out into the sunlight of spirit. Be grateful that you have come to the root of a particular thorny issue. Finally letting it go may prove tricky as you find the ego part of you wants to hold onto this fight. See it for what it is: the ego self. Give yourself a talking to if required: do I really want to continue to colour my life through this attachment, bringing me down and thwarting my spiritual progress? Have the courage to hand it over to Divine Mother who is silently waiting and to receive Her blessings. You have the free choice to hold on and ultimately suffer some more or let go and be free.

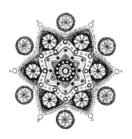

In this chapter, I teach a method of chipping away the dross to reveal the shining you within through a *kriya* (cleansing) breath called *Ujjayi*. There are many battles to be waged with the ego as soon as one sits to meditate. The first battle is waged with the senses to withdraw the consciousness inward. *Ujjayi*, meaning 'victorious' or 'to conquer', is a rasping breath focused through a slightly open but restricted throat which helps gain victory over ego consciousness. It builds great spiritual strength for all its simplicity to execute. You may like to think of the physical grossness of the body residing within the torso and limbs. In lifting the consciousness from the body through the narrowing of the body of the neck, placing awareness in the breath, there is a process of cathartic alchemy, from the consciousness residing in the grosser elements (base chakra, earth; sacral chakra, water; navel chakra, fire; heart chakra, air) through the narrowing of the throat to the subtle element ether, in the throat chakra.

Ujjayi is very beneficial for those suffering from asthma as it opens the airways to work more efficiently. It gives you a warrior-like focus to chisel away that which you are not.

In the initial stage, *Ujjayi* involves awareness of the natural breath without trying to influence breathing ratio. It involves a concentration on the rasping sound of the breath heard in a slightly constricted throat during inhalation and exhalation. In a later stage, one introduces pauses between inhale and exhale/exhale and inhale (*kumbhaka*). With total awareness on the sensation and sound of the breath in the throat, the mind starts to relax and expand into a feeling of tranquillity.

As one starts to master this shift in consciousness from physical to more subtle awareness, one starts to move prana (life force) itself. This is experienced as a stream of pure white light or as a trickling or burning sensation in the chest or throat.

Pranayama: The *Ujjayi* (Victory) Breath

Sit upright for meditation. Close the eyes and become aware of the regularity of the breath.

Be aware of the breath as it passes through the nostrils as a sensation of coolness with the inhale and warmth with the exhale. Try to just observe the breath without interrupting the flow. Watch as the breath settles into a longer, slower, more relaxed rhythm: cool on the inhale; warm on the exhale.

Transfer awareness to the sound and/or sensation of the breath in the throat.

Keep the lips together and gently let the jaw open slightly. Notice the shift in the sound of the breath as you do so.

Next try to slightly constrict the throat so that a soft snoring sound is heard in the throat. It can be felt as a more obvious sensation of air passing through the throat. Imagine that you are breathing from the throat, not the nostrils.

Try to have the face relaxed. The throat constriction is only slight so that you can maintain it continuously throughout and should not bring any discomfort. Allow the breath to become long, slow and controlled: the slower the better. Keep focusing on the soft sound in the throat which should be only audible to you.

There is no prescription on the count of the breath or on any pauses which may naturally develop as the sense of tranquillity deepens. Just be conscious of a long, slow breath in the throat. The body may hold the *prana* gathered from the inhale or after the exhale, if so, just focus the pause on the brow.

The body may experience the Breathless State: an absence of needing to breathe. If so, stay with the peacefulness of the breathless state. Just enjoy the calmness as the body will breathe again when it needs to.

Through the simplest of breaths, the *ujjayi*, you become clean. All temporary grafts on the beauty of your soul are chiselled away through the simplicity of the breath.

Practise for 5 minutes.

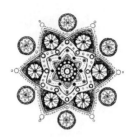

The focus of the meditation on Cleansing Power of Peace is to chisel away temporary blemishes on the perfection of your soul to reveal who you truly are. In so doing, you step up to become a manufacturer of peace in the world, emanating peace to all beings.

Meditation: Cleansing Power of Peace

Prayer: *Divine Spirit, chisel Thou my life. Draw Thy Divine elixir from the grossness of my frame. Reveal Thy light, reveal Thy peace and reveal Thyself within my heart. Om Shanti Peace.*

Sitting with the spine straight for meditation, shift the weight from left to right until your consciousness becomes centred in the spine.

Become aware of the level of the eyes. Above and between the eyes is the *ajna* (brow) chakra as a disc of light. Be aware of the body breathing in the head so that you can feel the breath.

Take awareness to the nostrils and notice the body breathing without trying to influence the length or quality of the breath.

There is awareness of the breath blowing behind the eyes and coolness across the brain with the inhale. And a warmth rippling over the brain with the exhale. Just notice.

Allow the awareness of breath to come down into the throat. Start the *Ujjayi* breath. Watch the body breathe in and out with a rasping sound in the throat.

There is a beauty in the inhale, perhaps holding that beauty on the brow and a soft letting go, blowing away from the body as you breathe out, manufacturing peace around the body.

Stay with the process of the *ujjayi* breath, dissolving your awareness into the breath. Stay with the wonder and magic of that as if you didn't want to blink and miss it.

Pull back on the effort of *ujjayi* so that it is much softer and maintain it for 10 minutes. The *ujjayi* breath is chiselling away what you are not to reveal what you are.

If attention wanders, just bring it back to the sensation of the breath in the throat, before moving back into subtlety again.

Become like an atmosphere processor manufacturing peace. Breath by breath, that which is not at peace within is transmuted into peace. (Just place your attention in the breath and let it do its work, rather than pondering what may be transmuted.)

The consciousness starts to rise in the spine. It comes with an experience of 'headiness' but stay with the sensation of the breath. As the consciousness rises up through each of the chakras, it may come with signature awareness or tastes in the throat.

Just stay with the breath. Breathe in 'beauty' of the breath through the throat. With a pause after the inhale, rest 'beauty' on the brow which is transferred into calmness in the brain.

When you have gathered beauty and calmness on the brow, the exhale breathes that beauty through the pores of the skin, like many little flames.

The body becomes a dotted outline as beauty and calmness are breathed out through many little pores. Each little flame chips off another aspect of that which you are not.

Perhaps your *ujjayi* breath has become very subtle, almost inaudible. (Keep coming back to the sensation of the breath if that is what is helping you to be anchored in the consciousness of this meditation.)

Rest Calmness on the brow, amplify it and then exhale it through the pores of the skin as peace flames. Perhaps your peace flames are tiny flickers, as points of light. Perhaps they are great rays of light in all directions.

Mentally repeat the mantra: *I am Peace. Peace blows through the pores of my body into infinity.*

Experience yourself as a radiance of peace without boundaries, across all space. As the internal expands to become external, the divine elixir of your life spark is One with the Great Ocean of Life.

Use the mantra to purify, not only your body but your whole environment, your town, your nation and the planet. Become a living, breathing manufacturer of peace on the Earth.

Finish with the prayer: *Divine Spirit, Reveal Thy light, reveal Thy peace within my heart. And let me give that peace to all. Om Shanti Peace.*

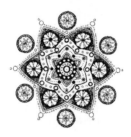

With this practice you can learn to do battle with those aspects of habit which are unhelpful and to develop a peace-filled practice in everyday living. You can tread with peaceful movements and peaceful breaths, visualising that you are moving within that expanded bubble of peace. This practice not only changes yourself but it changes those that you meet and the world around you as you become a spiritual being manufacturing peace as you operate in a physical world.

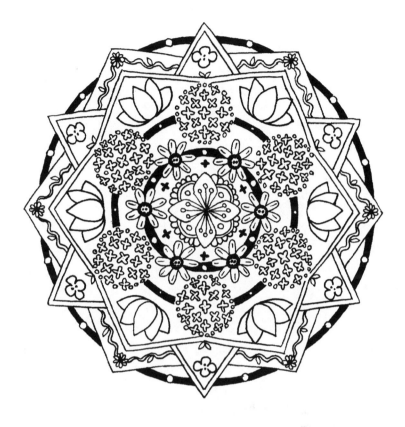

Chapter 12

Awakening the Lotus of Peace

There is a beautiful inner garden of heavenly peace just waiting to be discovered. In order to awaken the lotus of peace within, we must learn to rise above the ego consciousness. Meditation is the route of withdrawing from entrapment in the allure of *maya* to awaken to our true reality as the unlimited, eternal soul. Above the clouds, the sun is always shining. Even on the gloomiest day, when the aeroplane of our consciousness rises clear of the clouds, we discover just how sunny and peaceful it is.

In this chapter, we are learning to attune to the lotus of light in the crown chakra (*sahasara*) and lift our consciousness above the cloudy waters of *maya*, to keep our mind steady and focused on overcoming all distractions in life. We can mentally have our consciousness in being 'above' the narrative of our personal drama. Imagine that you are the lotus of peace, with your lotus head shining above the doom and gloom. That is the way to rise above being subject to *avidya* (individual delusion) and *maya* (cosmic delusion).

Nature is the cause of our apparent separateness. God created nature but under a camouflage of delusion. We are pure spirit hidden in the covering of a physical body and that leads to our appearance of being apart from spirit. We may think that we make free choices in acting in this world but we are subject to the laws of nature which influence the choices that we make. That is, the three *gunas*: *sattva, rajas* and *tamas* (see Chapter 7). As humans, we, like the animal kingdom, are subject to the bounds of the laws of nature, except that animals act purely from instinctual responses to nature and we have the *potential* to use our free will to break free from instinctual habitual responses. But do we? How many times are we drawn to repeat 'safe' habits, such as a certain route from A to B? A certain order for ablutions in the morning? A practised habit of addressing and reacting to others? How present and aware are we in the mundanities of daily life? How much of our daily actions are mindless, reactionary habits and how much are truly chosen with our free will from free choice? With our lifespan of 60–80 years, how much are we different from the animals? Within the heart of every being, plant, animal or human, resides a soul which is a microcosmic reflection of the Great Spirit, but that soul light is obscured by the Cosmic Delusion within the covering of a physical form that breathes, being either rooted as in plants or with the power of locomotion, with innate instinctual tendencies or with the power of free will. Although most humans would like to think that they have totally free will, an examination of their actions reveals that they are in fact tied to habit, instinct and reaction, not unlike the animal kingdom. Only when we are self-aware do we chart beyond the confines of nature and truly act from free will.

We do, however, have free choice. Our free choice in *how* we respond in any scenario from *tamas* (dense selfishness, ignorance, sluggishness), *rajas* (either acting from self-interest or acting to free the soul) or *sattva* (acting for the good of others) is influenced by and dictated by how high we have evolved as a soul in spiritual consciousness. There is a corresponding weight of karma, whether we use that freedom of choice to act from habit or in fully-conscious awareness.

The spiritual progress demonstrated on the scale of spiritual evolution of how far we have journeyed from mindless habit and reactions to soul-consciousness is mapped out in the ladder of our astral spine. Although we may have evolved through meditation, until we have eliminated and overcome all *samskaras* (seed tendencies from our past or present lives), we may find an old reaction popping up as a harbouring of one of the *doshas* (faults of the ego) which causes us to react *tamasically*. Subject to our personal *avidya* (delusion), we like to think that we have eliminated all layers, threads and seeds of *samskara* in one sitting, but that presumption is also another of the ego's delusions. Try to be unsurprised and undisturbed at anything that arises from within: just keep meditating and handing over any hint of reaction that comes to your attention. Over a period of time, any reactions which are still harboured by the ego become more and more subtle: no more big storm clouds and wailing dramas. These are cleared, which allows whispers of disgruntled moods, shadows of selfish thoughts or wisps of wishing harm to others to come into focus. Treat all *samskaras* (temporary blemishes on your otherwise perfect soul) alike, with a welcome, for each one that is revealed to your attention is another obstacle potentially removed from your spiritual path. All such 'visitors' are the same, no matter how pleasant or unpleasant. Just as good moods are a result of good karma in the past, bad moods are a result of bad karma. Treat moods all the same, with indifference. Seek to get behind all these moves to seek He who made you and therein find all comfort, harmony, happiness and joy that you long for. Through good karma and meditation, we gradually ascend the spiritual path and our seat of consciousness rises higher and higher in the spine.

We are learning to think and act consciously beyond the constraints of habit under the influence of the *gunas*. You could analyse yourself and determine if you are on the upward evolutionary scale according to nature (the slow route of spiritual progress), or generally on the downward evolutionary scale in blind thinking under the thrall of reactive emotions, or whether you are forthrightly taking the fast route by persevering with yoga and meditation which progress is evidenced in your successful translation of the soul qualities of peace, forgiveness, love and compassion into your daily life.

At times, my students have some conflict between acting unselfishly for the benefit of others, such as household chores or charitable acts, and being 'selfish' in absenting oneself in order to meditate. It should be noted here that choosing to take time out from daily duties to meditate is not a selfish act. It is our inherent God-given duty to seek Him who made us and to rise above the circumstances in which He placed us. Meditation and quiet are a necessary route to that awakening in God-consciousness, the whole reason why we are in incarnation. Therefore, God's laws override the lesser responsibilities of us humans. In meditating to seek God, there is no karma. Quite the opposite, through elevating our consciousness in meditation, old bad karma is being quietly erased.

Don't get too caught up in the actions that you make in daily life. Who is it that acts? You may think that it is you who acts but, sadly, that is the deluded ego talking. The deeper that you progress in meditation, the more you realise that many of those actions which we took to be chosen in free will are actually the habits of body-identified ego, subject to the laws of nature (the three *gunas*). So, who is it that acts? If all our body, powers, thoughts and even our free will are borrowed from God, then it must be really He who acts. When you lift your arm, God provided the body, the power of movement and the free will to 'think' that you move it. All life circumstances, possessions, even the people in your life are all borrowed: you do not own any of them. So, who, in any one instance, is acting?

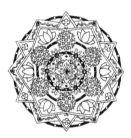

The following exercise is an introspection to discover how much your 'free will' is dictated to by upward evolutionary good vibrations from nature or from even higher soul impulses as a result of practising meditation and good karma, or by downward evolutionary bad vibrations from delusive habituation to natural influences (subject to nature through the three *gunas*) and bad karma.

Exercise: Introspection on Free Will

Am I meditating every day?

How deeply do I meditate? (Do I skim the surface or do I dive deeply?) Depth may vary depending on what you are facing in your personal challenges, but aim to make each day deeper than the last.

Am I beset with bad moods? Do I have changeable moods? Any mood which is the result of having a sense-pleasure gratified, even if it is a good mood, is still a mood. Aim to overcome all moodiness. Moods are the ego's domain, like the dark, muddy waters of the lake in which the lotus bulb is planted. The lotus must grow up from the depths, through dark, silty water to open out into the health-giving blessings of the sunlight of spirit.

How much am I habit-bound, like a hamster on a treadmill? How often do I break free and choose to forge a new path? Am I scared of change? You might experiment with taking another route through the park or shaking up the order in which you usually do proceedings. Aim to have at least one moment a day when you break the mould, challenge yourself or think outside the box.

Am I operating through selfish actions? Unselfish actions? Which of the three modes of nature am I operating through? Note that it is very tiring in the heart when you operate through the ego.

Explore your inclinations to think or act in a certain way. When we awaken to the sunlight of the soul, we realise that God is the performer of all actions, not our unpredictable ego-separateness.

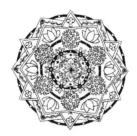

We learn to be undisturbed by the seeming ups and downs of this world of duality, to take it all with a pinch of salt. To relish every moment, awake in the sunlight of God, we must be awake in the intuitive understanding of the higher states of consciousness. A poor ego-bound person is never happy. A person awake in soul-consciousness on the other hand is always supremely happy, be he in a palace, the humblest abode, alone or in a crowd, being born or at bodily death, change does not shake his happiness. Evolving on a path of meditation and spiritual growth will inexorably lead us to a state of unshakeable calm in all circumstances, unaffected by the changeable influences of nature. To be incarnated in a body, one must take on some of the constraints of the delusive physical world but when we persevere in going within to meditate casting aside all burdens, including the body, to sit in the quiet within, there all truths will be revealed to you. Seek and you will find that you are fully awake in the arms of the Divine.

Whether we like it or not, until we are awake, we are being driven by one of the qualities of nature at any one time. *Sattva*, the highest quality, is operating from the higher chakras at the throat, brow and crown (although strictly speaking the crown, *sahasrara*, is not a chakra but a state of becoming) in an attitude of peace, love and benevolence. The lower three chakras, base, sacral and navel, are operating under *tamas*, which is alternating between moods, unhappiness, inertia, boredom, unwillingness to make change and emotional outbursts in reaction to what life throws. In the centre, operating at heart level, is the activating principle of *rajas*, which provides the propulsion to operate from *tamas*, selfishness or *sattva*, unselfishness. It is the heart that provides the driving impetus to either of these opposites: actively selfish or actively unselfish.

One may discern one's stage of spiritual development and karmic clarity or density by gazing at the spiritual eye in meditation. In the brow chakra, seen with astral sight, there is a triangle symbolising the three *gunas*. The predominance of one or other of these three qualities will glow: white in the top point shows a predominance of *sattva*, or the left point will glow red, indicating *rajasistic* predominance or the right will be dark, indicating *tamas* is temporarily dominant. Only when all three points glow equally does that indicate the perfect balance: *tamas* is needed to maintain the physical body and hold the atoms together, *rajas* is needed to activate the body, drawing power for all physical functions from the astral realms and *sattva* is needed to steer the consciousness towards right-discriminating wisdom. We overcome the three states of nature, not by 'fighting them' but by being undisturbed by whatever arises, as in the Buddhist practice of dispassion.

The battlefield of life is waged on three fronts which mirror the three modes of nature. The surface of the skin and deep tissue of the body is the realm of *tamas* which seeks to collude with the ego in keeping us bound to sensory pleasure and stimulation. On succeeding to withdraw the consciousness out of the tissue of the body and the senses, we move into the second battlefield which is in the spine. The spine is the abode of the activating principle, *rajas* with its downward current *apana* under the thrall of the ego to be downwardly devolving in consciousness or the upward current of *prana* to be upwardly evolving and the control of the soul. On claiming victory in the other two battlefields, one gains the third battlefield in the brain as the soul seeks to turn within for the answers to its origin or to be outwardly focused. This is the realm of *sattva*.

This, then, is the battle which you must face as you go within to meditate each day. Having been victorious over the ego yesterday in winning control of the senses and withdrawal of consciousness into the heart (winning a place on the second battlefield), you may find that what was easily won the previous day is an uphill struggle as you close your eyes and prepare to go within. It may be an intense effort to even claim square one today. This moveable, changeable feast of experience is the result of past *karma* and *samskaras* that are carried within, cloaking the light of the soul. So be prepared to do battle as you still the body for meditation. Until you have dissolved all blocks to your spiritual progress, the daily battle to retain concentration to side with the soul is an unpredictable quantity. You may find three days of battle wins you a day or two of joy as you flow within in meditation. Or there may be a week of battling for even the smallest incremental progress. Or conversely, there may be weeks of being enveloped in peace and bliss as you meditate. Show up each day without expectation: just because it has been a struggle/easy the previous day is no indication that it will be the same today. But show up for meditation anyway. Therein lies the secret of progressing spiritually through meditation-perseverance, diligence and practice.

You are making spiritual progress, although the ladder of progression may at times be two steps forward and three steps back, never doubt that you are succeeding. The general level of spiritual acumen that we have reached and maintain in daily life, is evidenced by open and clear lotus chakras. The root of each of the seven main chakras in the astral spine is the source of subtle streamers of astral light which appear as 'petals'. Each chakra (meaning 'wheel' or 'disc') is perceived as a vibrating flower of shimmering light. Whether a chakra is open, closed or partially open is determined by any remaining debris that still shrouds its astral light and impedes its healthful functioning. Even without astral sight, a blocked chakra is evidenced by tightness, feeling closed off, unfeeling, remote, afraid or unconsciously shielding the body by folding the arms (navel chakra) or wearing a scarf (throat chakra) etc. The solution to all partially functioning chakras is practice Alternate Nostril Breath (*nadi shodhanam*), pray and meditate deeply. Don't worry overly much. Just discern and keep up your daily meditation practice as the panacea of all ills.

The evolutionary journey through the spine back to Spirit is mapped on the spine. In the following preliminary meditation, we access the super-conscious awareness to view the spine indicating our present level of spiritual evolution.

Meditation: The Spinal Ladder of Spiritual Progress

Prayer: *Divine Father, Loving Mother, awaken my intuitive perception that I may know that I live by Thy grace. Let the sunshine of Thy wisdom awaken within me. Om Shanti Peace.*

Be aware of the body breathing either side of an upright spine.

Visualise the spine as a column of light with red at base chakra, orange, yellow, pale blue at the base of the throat, deep blue at the back of the head and pure white thousand-petalled lotus above the head.

Watch the currents of light within the spine as you breathe – there is a slight upward movement of *prana* with the inhale and a downward movement of *apana* with the exhale.

There is calmness with the in-breath and a settling back to the base as you breathe out.

Focus the two currents of the physical eyes on the brow. Visualise the spiritual eye on the brow as a bright moon of light until it gets brighter and brighter.

From the viewpoint of the middle of the head, gaze down the ladder of light into the spine.

Where has your level of consciousness risen to?

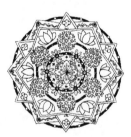

The results of this exercise will be different over time as you are constantly evolving to Spirit. During the course of a meditation your conscious level will rise in the spine especially if you sit for longer periods or dive deeply. However, the real litmus test of each spiritual rung attained is: Can I maintain this level of consciousness, of peace, joy and harmony in the pressing duties of everyday living? It is normal for that level, like mercury in a thermometer, to drop after your meditation but gradually we restructure our battery to hold greater charge, i.e., we learn how to effectively contain this level of *prana*-light as we function physically in the world.

All distortions of *maya* disappear with the awakening of soul realisation. As moonlight is refracted into a million shattered reflections when water is agitated, the pure reflection as a shining disc of light comes back into focus as the water returns to stillness. In meditation, we allow the perfume of soul consciousness to rise above the ego delusions and *maya*, like oil on water to behold the perfection of the mooned face of the soul. Imagine that you could rise above that lake of duality and fly free. There are so many bright blooms of distraction that might take your interest but you learn to keep your awareness on the sunlight of soul consciousness. Lesser attractions then lose their allure and what seemed as bright lustre is finally perceived as dull, tarnished and hollow. While in incarnation in a physical body, we bridge two realms, the physical and the spiritual. In super-conscious meditation, we realise that we can act *in* the world using free will while at the same time maintaining the expansive super-conscious awareness that you are not *of* the world.

In the Awakening the Lotus of Peace Meditation, we rise above mortal consciousness and become the thousand-petalled lotus (*crown chakra* or astral brain), offering our uniquely exquisite perfume as a gift to the Divine.

Meditation: Awakening the Lotus of Peace

Visualise that upright column of light in the spine from the base to the crown of the head.

Prayer: *Divine Spirit, let me be a radiant flower in Thy Infinite garden, or a tiny star ornamenting the vastness of Thy heavens, or the humblest place within Thy heart. Om Shanti Peace.*

Behind the eyelids, focus the eyes to look slightly up to a single point of the brow.

Breathe in for a count of 6 and breathe out for a count of 6. Aim for a clear calmness in the head as you breathe. Imagine that you are breathing in the cool calmness of a mountain stream.

Breathe in and out from the same count (if 6 is too short, breathe in and out for a count of 8).

Take your attention from the front of the body and recede back into the spine. Visualise the astral spine and the *brahma nadi* (pathway to God), the super-fine causal spine, superimposed on the physical spine.

Visualise that you are in that column of light from the base of the spine up to the crown as you continue to breathe in and out for a count of 6 (or 8). Incorporate a pause after the inhale and hold the attention at the crown during the pause (no count, just hold the awareness).

Imagine the brilliant white petals of the thousand-petalled lotus radiating pure white light from each of its thousand petals.

Breathe in for a count of 6 (or 8), awareness rises up the spine. Hold the awareness in the pause at the thousand-petalled lotus. Breathe out for a count of 6 (or 8), awareness floats back down the spine.

Imagine the radiation of light from the crown-lotus in all directions: upward, behind, in front, left, right and down through the body.

Replace the mental count with the mental mantra *So Ham*: Inhale mentally saying *So*, hold the breath and awareness at the crown, exhale mentally saying *Ham*. Allow your attention to be in the mantra (the breath is only the vehicle).

Visualise the crown as a pure white lotus sitting on the surface of a deep pool of water. The base chakra is rooted in the deep silt at the bottom of the pool. The other chakras are strung out along the stem as it rises to the crown, floating on the surface as a lotus of light above the surface of *maya* (duality, illusion).

Your consciousness is above the water of *maya*, radiating pure white light in all directions from your lotus of light.

Rise above the dark waters of *maya* (illusion) into the sunlight of spirit as you awaken to your true soul consciousness.

There is only light. The darkness is behind.

As the lotus of light, you are filled with the perfume of peace. Peace exudes as a perfume from each one of your thousand beautiful petals.

Each petal is a perfect ray of light, exuding the most beautiful and unique perfume to produce a symphony of scent. Exquisite and pure, bathe in the scent of your own perfume.

Visualise your beautiful heart chakra with its lotus of light rotating upward in the spine to lend its light and beauty to the crown lotus of light.

Visualise that the beautiful petals on the throat chakra rotate to face the crown chakra, lending the light of its 16 petals to the crown. All the chakras in the spine rotate upward to face the crown, their lights flowing upwards into the crown. The lotus of light above the head becomes brighter and brighter across an ocean of sky and the scent increases. Bathe in the exquisite perfume of the crown, more beautiful than any rose.

Look down into the spine, you can see the light from each chakra flowing upward: red petals of the base chakra, orange petals of the sacrum, yellow of the navel pointing upwards, heart in green, pit of the throat in pale blue pointing upward. The chakras are a garden of flowers within your own being.

Your scent is unique, the essence of your soul. As every snowflake is unique, so your essence is unique within creation.

The body inhales, breathe in your scent, offering that scent as a gift to the divine with the exhale.

Experience or imagine that perfume rising up from within as you breathe in and offering that essence with the out-breath. The more that you concentrate on your uniqueness as a soul, the more your perfume will arise from within.

Offer your scent as if you were laying it on the altar of the divine.

Affirmation: *I lay the Perfume of Peace from my soul at the feet of the Divine.*

Offering your highest essence, your light, your perfume, you evoke a response from the Divine. Receiving the perfume of the Divine into each one of your chakra blossoms so there is both an offering and a receiving. That perfume is both exuding from your own being and blowing directly from the Divine, blowing through you: harmonious, loving and kind.

Direction has no meaning. There is only here, now, everywhere.

Prayer: *Divine Father, Divine Mother, awaken my intuitive perception that I may know that I live and act by Thy Grace. Let the sunshine of Thy wisdom awaken within me, awaken within me. Om Shanti Peace.*

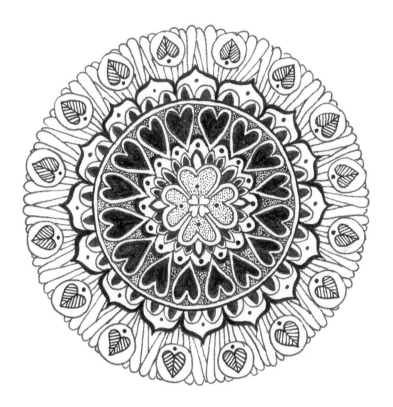

Chapter 13

The Divine Elixir of Peace

Peace is the essential nature of the soul. Worldly activity leads us away from an inner calm to constant agitation; always busy with this or that. There is hardly a moment when one activity is completed before another one begins. We may watch the busy ant going about his business and marvel at his industriousness, moving mountains of sand or objects which far outweigh his body mass. His short lifespan is full of nonstop motion until death overcomes him. Are our lives like the ant's?

The busyness of the world intrudes in our potential peace if we open to it. Each activity sets up a fresh ripple on the surface of our peace. All day long, one ripple after another disturbs and erodes our calm. But surely, if we are divine beings, is a way to enact in the world without feeling that our inner peace is fraught and fractured? Once we are in tune with it, is there a way to contain our precious vessel of soul peace? In this chapter, we explore the three *gunas* (modes of nature) and how to balance activity while at the same time maintaining the inner calm of the soul.

Until we are liberated from ceaseless incarnations, we are subject to the law of karma. As a being bound to repeated incarnation, we are continually operating through one of the three modes of nature (*gunas*): *tamas, rajas* and *sattva*. We are subject to acting in this world and in so doing, operating the heart energy (*rajas* – constant activity) through one of the other two qualities, which are: acting from selfish motives to our benefit alone (*tamas – dark or ignorant*) or acting from a benevolent motive that seeks the benefit of others (*sattva – good or unselfish*). The massive generator in the heart is the neutral quality which gives us the energy to act selfishly or unselfishly in the world. You know the saying that *his heart wasn't in it.* In harnessing the motivation of the heart, we open to the full potential of energy that we can tap from the divine source through the magnet of the heart chakra.

As long as we are subjected to the laws of karma and tied to the wheel of continued incarnation, to be in the world is to act. We must act: eat, cater for the body's needs, interact with others and seek to free ourselves from soul bondage. Even breathing is an action. If we are not to be like a hamster on a treadmill, we must seek the path that all good-seeking souls, saints and masters have trodden before us.

The huge generator of the heart is key. We are only accessing a tiny fraction of the huge potential of the heart to bring about change on this planet. The greatest service that we can do is to change ourselves, to realise our divine nature. How do we awaken to our full heart potential? How can we act in the world while at the same time holding onto our soul's purpose in being here?

God watches the heart. Nothing is hidden from God, no act of kindness, prayers for others, grimy little secret or unkind act is hidden. In the eyes of God, we are transparent. The heart is the true indicator of your state of being, either selfish or unselfish. Think of your motivations for performing any action.

By way of illustration, I'd like to share an incident from my childhood. I had a white mouse which escaped into the garden. My brother and sister were trying to help me catch this wayward mouse, but it was like lightning. It was running along the garden wall and my brother had thwarted its exit by placing a plank of wood at right angles to the wall. The mouse turned about and darted in the opposite direction. Quickly, I rammed another plank of wood against the wall... just as the mouse reached it. The poor thing was squashed, gave a squeak and died. I had killed it. I felt remorseful but was consoled by the knowledge that I had been trying to save the mouse as it would not have lasted a night at large. What was the greater karma that I accrued with this act: to act and inadvertently cause harm or to avoid acting and leave the mouse to an uncertain fate? Does the *intention* to help or harm have influence on the weight of karma? The guidance of the Bhagavad Gita is very clear in this matter. There are degrees of karma: good (*sattvic*) actions incur less karma than bad (*tamasic*) actions.

God watches the intentions of our heart, *behind* the actions themselves. As you sow so shall you reap. God watches the secret motivations behind why we act. The ego is very pernicious and comes up with all sorts of reasons as to why or how you could appear to be goodie-two-shoes. Be prepared to look honestly behind the acts themselves to the underlying intention. I'm sure that most of us will have refined our actions to benevolent ones but look for the intentions behind them as the ego is very subtle in seeking to have satisfaction for the little self (the ego).

As you sow so shall you reap. There are degrees of karma

but it is still a balance which must be redressed at some time in the future, either this lifetime or the next. Be honest with yourself and bring your intentions out into the cold, hard light of discernment.

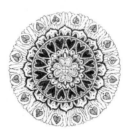

Exercise: Reflection on the Intentions behind My Actions

Sit quietly with an upright spine and closed eyes for a few moments. Watch the breath until you come into a place of calm.

Think of a mundane action, such as cleaning or mowing the lawn, which you did today, yesterday or are about to do. Look at the action to the intention behind it. Is there perhaps a secret intention to gain some reward or attention for doing that activity? (I'm a good boy because I do... or I'm a good girl because I....)

Am I being open and kind to others for the right reasons? Or do I harbour a longing for recognition, acclaim or praise?

Am I acting while in a state of anger, secretly blaming another or seeking to prove a point?

Do I have any weeds of selfishness to pull out of the divine garden of my heart?

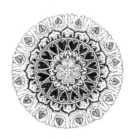

Anahata, the heart chakra, is in the centre of the seven main chakras. It has the potential to be balanced, like the centre point in a pair of balance scales. At some point in your spiritual evolution, the heart chakra will rotate to face upward in the spine thereby releasing its magnetic power to the astral brain, *sahasrara*, the highest chakra. Any little mar or selfishness held within the heart chakra will be exposed in stark view as an area of darkness which can feel tight or dense. Sri Yukteswar Giri, the guru of Paramahansa Yogananda, described the process of evolving from a human being to a divine being in five transformative stages of the heart from a dark heart (closed, harbouring dark deeds, selfish intentions) to a clear heart (open, transparent, guileless, truthful, loving).

Meditation: Peace within the Heart

Sit upright and allow the breath to settle. Make your own heartfelt prayer.

Lift the hands. Balance left and right as if weighing the hands – is one heavier than the other? Let go of any perceived weight.

Bring the heels of the thumbs together in praying hands gesture at the sternum. Tune into the quality of the breath, like listening to the steady rhythm of a child breathing.

Bring heel of thumbs to the brow and bridge of the nose.

Breathe in an unhurried breath for a count of four. Hold awareness on the bridge of the nose (hold the peace), breathe out for a count of four.

Return the heels of hands to the heart. Hold the attention here in reverence of the peace within the heart (at first this will be blind faith until, before long, this can be felt and experienced as expansive cosmic peace).

Repeat bridging peace between the brow and the heart, amplifying the frequency of peace.

One point of note is that in order to act from a peaceful

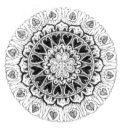

heart, it doesn't necessarily mean that we should try to please others all the time. Sometimes, it would serve others better if you spoke the truth rather than trying to please them. If one is acting to avoid being out of favour, then fear is the motivation of that act, not love. Maintain your integrity to hold onto your principles. Be vigilant that pride or envy are not holding court in your heart.

Even benevolent acts incur some karma if they have any intention of personal gain or finding satisfaction from the fruits of the actions. Weed out any selfish motivation in the heart as you spiritually evolve from a dark heart, which holds on to desire for personal gain, to a clear heart. To evolve into the clear heart, every action is offered to God and the intention behind each action is only to please God. Only those wholly unselfish actions incur no karma. An act could be a mundane task, such as washing a dish or mowing the lawn, but these are excellent repetitive tasks with which to practise dissociation from the ego. You learn to act, not from ego gain or worldly acclaim, but solely to please God.

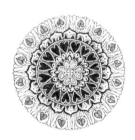

Exercise: Practising the Mindful Art of Dishwashing

Select a dish. Practise mindfully washing the dish.

Allow the dish to be the centre of your world to the exclusion of all else as if this item were a most cherished priceless heirloom.

Really look at the item, as if seeing it for the first time.

Be in the Now.

Will I have any personal benefit in having a clean dish? Watch how the mind jumps into a future where you are using the dish.

Pull it back into the present moment. Mentally hand over any benefit that you may accrue from the clean dish.

Practise the action of washing the dish as a gift to the Divine. Act solely to please God.

Notice any attachment to acting for personal gain, even in mundane tasks. Practise handing over all ego attachments. (Even that little intention of having a clean dish to eat from, is ego attachment to the result of your action and will accrue some karma. But in handing over an action, however simple, there is no karma.)

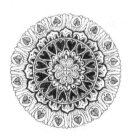

It is good to practise dissolving attachment to gain from the results of our actions. It is good to practise renouncing selfish reasons for acting as a mindfulness exercise on simple, mundane actions. In solitary tasks that you may do frequently, you can commandeer these as learning tools to practise renunciation, in short, achievable 'bites'. That is how you move towards a clear heart: one act of renunciation after another.

Remember that our power of volition and locomotion, this body, mind and soul, all come from God. We have borrowed that power to eat, breathe, think, imagine and feel: everything comes from God and is God. Through the technique of meditation, we wake from our selfish ego-desire-led motivations and one by one hand the action *and* the result (benefit) from the action to God (who is really the actor here). In ignorance of the truth, we foolishly think it is I (the ego) who thinks, moves and operates this body. That blinkered 'reality' is the maya (illusion) world of the ego, looking out through its dream-clouded web of thoughts and desires into that murky dream-world that we call earth. In waking from this dream, through repeatedly striving in meditation and acting to please God, we realise that this world is nothing but a matrix of energy and intelligent patterning of *prana* (life force) dreamed by God. In microcosm, every cell of our body is an energy-*prana* patterning within a complex relationship with all the other cells to operate as a homogenous whole, communicating with each other, interdependent and constantly replacing old cells with new ones so that the whole functions well as a learning-vehicle for the lifetime of one soul: you. It is remarkable to contemplate how perfectly functioning this intelligent body is, without the need for conscious effort on your part. The intelligent energy matrix of your body was gifted by God so that you can incarnate on the dream-world of earth with a fresh opportunity to forsake all the errors of the ego-led ways and choose of your own free will to turn your back on earthly toys and to come back into your true home in spirit. In reality, you, the soul, is ever-awake in deepest joy, at one with God, you just don't fully 'know' that yet.

The problem for souls in incarnation, in the murky darkness of illusion, is that we forget our home in spirit. Except that in our heart there is a longing for something wonderful that we know we have lost. That secret longing to know God and be One is with us quietly yearning, silently urging us to return, no matter how many millennia of lifetimes we tarried distracted by the glittering sham of the physical world. For all it promises (if I only had... I would be happy), satisfaction is never the permanent result of any desire. Each desire leads the ego-bound consciousness down winding pathways, like a musk deer forever seeking the source of that delightful perfume, never to realise that the ecstatic source of the fragrance is its own self. Ego + desire = attachment and karmic consequences. Such is the lesson of earthly living. Wake up, sleeping beauty!

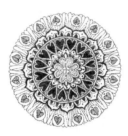

Prana is the universal building block underlying quarks, electrons and atoms, existing throughout the whole of creation as a field of vibrating energy. That *prana* is in every cell of the body, the air we breathe, sunlight, water and the food that we eat. It is constantly changing as we consume and discharge *prana* by the way that we interact with the environment around us. That is, how we act, what we say and how we think all have a bearing on whether we receive or leak *prana*. Eventually, we evolve spiritually by learning that stray unkind remarks, unkind thoughts or acting through anger, will drain that inner reservoir of peace and of *prana*. Fortunately, by tapping into the universal source of life through yoga breathing (*pranayama*) and meditation, we replenish from the limitless supply of cosmic *prana*.

In the following meditation, aim to go deeper in stages: focus on moving into the breath, away from the body; then into mantra and away from the breath; thirdly, let the mantra lift your consciousness to a highly elevated vibration. Try to resist any urge to move the body as physical movement sets up a restless vibration which draws consciousness out of the developing stillness.

You may have periods when the breath slows to an almost imperceptible suggestion of breathing or stops. In these periods of 'breathlessness' you are being sustained by the direct stream of divine life force (*prana*) that is flowing through you, and not by air. The body has expelled all toxins and no longer needs to breathe for these moments. This is a deeper stage of going within (*pratyahara*) and is to be allowed, but not forced. Merely holding the breath is not the 'breathless state'. Try to observe and allow this state without ego interference.

Meditation: Receiving the Elixir of Peace

Sit upright for meditation and close the eyes. Bring hands together at the heart.

Once your body is comfortable but alert, aim to sit motionless.

Prayer: *Beloved mother, fill us with the wine of Thy blessing flowing continually; let us be open and receptive to Thy blessing, let us be opened like the rose to the blessings of Thy love, let us be truthful and loving for that is the opening and clarity of the heart. Be with us now and always. Om Peace Amen.*

Bring your attention to the breath and allow the exhale to become longer. Watch the movement of breathing as if watching another body breathe. (Try to divest consciousness from the ego-body.)

Note the quality of the breath. How smooth is the transit of air?

Observe that the body is breathing of its own accord, like a set of bellows. You are not that body. You are the observer of the breath.

How soft is the quality of the breath? How smooth are the inhale and exhale? Any restlessness of body, mind (*manas*) or feeling (*chitta*) in the heart will create a raggedness in the breath.

You are detached, mentally slightly outside the body, observing it breathing.

Just observe. As you do so, there is a shift of consciousness, from the conscious mind to the subconscious. Take care that this shift does not result in drowsiness which is characteristic of the subconscious mind. Aim to chart the course of your ship to the wide awake super-conscious mind, beyond the doldrums of the subconscious.

Start to incorporate the *So Ham* mental mantra into your observation of the breath. Mentally say *So* with the inhale and *Ham* with the exhale. By this stage the breath may have receded in intensity from your awareness, as if slightly dislocated from it. Try to retain that objectivity and place your consciousness more in the mantra. The in-breath instigates the start of *So* and the exhale is the indicator to start *Ham*. There is a tie to the body via the breath but the mantra is the vehicle with which to loosen that tie by reminding you of who you are.

If the mind wanders, just be patient and bring it back to the observation that the body breathing prompts the *So Ham* mantra. Perhaps you are aware of the *So Ham* mantra starting to float your consciousness above the blinkered consciousness of the body.

Try to extricate any ego involvement in manipulating the breath. Ego interference is a hindrance to moving beyond body consciousness.

Start to float the consciousness. Imagine the *So Ham* mantra is playing out over the smooth surface of water. Allow the mantra to lift your consciousness. If your breath has become very still, then perhaps your mantra has ceased.

Visualise the lotus bulb rooted in the deep muddy silt at the bottom of the lake. The purity of the lotus is opening to the sunlight of spirit on the surface of the water. The water represents *maya* (illusion) or earthly consciousness. You, the soul, are the lotus.

Visualise the heart chakra filled with light and life. Heart chakra rotates upward to face *sahasrara*, the thousand-petalled lotus, the astral sun.

Feel into the heart. How open does it feel?

Visualise the twelve petals of the heart opening to receive the divine wine of peace which is constantly flowing through all hearts. Be open to receive this elixir of light filled with divine consciousness.

Is any part of the heart harbouring a resistance or tightness to being open? Visualise plucking that 'weed' out of the heart and offering it into the light of the divine.

Float your consciousness up, beyond the earthly realm into a higher realm of being.

Visualise that you are standing before a shining white marble temple of light. Feel magnetically drawn to climb the seven steps leading up into the temple.

Step onto the first step, symbolic of moving beyond earthly life.

On the second step, let go of all weight of sin.

On the third step, let go of ego consciousness.

Moving onto the fourth step, find great calmness.

On the fifth step, find great peace descending.

On the sixth step, have great vision and clarity to see things from a heavenly perspective.

Lastly, step on the platform of the temple. There is a great shimmering stream of light from you, coming as iridescent rays of light from within the temple. You cannot see within.

As you step into this iridescent stream of rainbow light, multi-coloured rays wash you inside and out. There are hues of every colour: shimmering blues, violets, pearlescent colours, rainbow pinks, golds, silvers and colours which are indescribable in earthly words.

Step forward into another stream of pure white light, being washed from the crown of the head and feeling your hands and feet being cleansed.

Step forward into the temple itself. It has one structure in the centre: a great white marble altar on which a single living flame is burning. There is a great being, the master Jesus, standing behind the altar. He invites you to step forward and to lay down your burdens.

Such peace and love are emanating from the eyes and hands of Jesus. Receive His great blessing.

Hand over anything that you would like to release at this time. You may wish to speak directly to the Great Master, one who has mastered earthly consciousness and is overflowing with Christ Consciousness.

Jesus produces a chalice. 'If you drink of this chalice, you will thirst no more.' This chalice is filled with the elixir of Divine Happiness. Jesus asks you to shed any feeling of unworthiness and reminds you that you are a soul of light, as much as He is. He gently places the chalice to your lips.

One liquid drop of elixir flows past your lips and into your being, awakening the heart so that your soul light shines forth. This cosmic elixir flows through your being removing seeds of untruth and selfishness from the heart as if they had never been.

Receive the blessings of the Blessed Christ as he says, 'I will be with you now and always. You need only think of me as close and I am close.'

The Great Master gently fades from your view and you are left standing in the stillness of the temple. Absorb the elevated vibration of this astral temple before coming out into the sunlight of spirit once more. Step down into a vast vista of gardens, waterfalls, lakes and mountains, as far as the eye can see, all shimmering in the light of God.

Allow the astral realm to recede from your view. Realise that you are sustained in a vast ocean of peace. From this elevated space, observe that the elixir of peace flows through all hearts.

In your own time, gently let awareness of your physical body filter back into focus.

Om Shanti Peace.

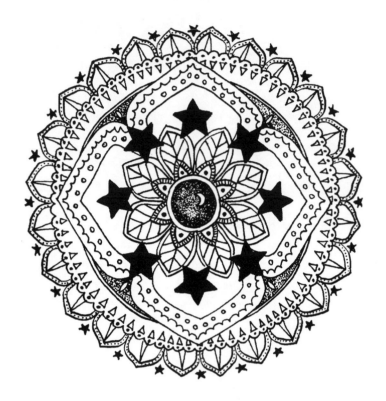

Chapter 14

The Stillness of Peace

Be still and know that I am God.
Psalm 46:10

We can make marvellous progress in meditation but still find
the ultimate goal of finding the Peace-God eludes us in daily life
if we are unrestrained in our emotions or become overwhelmed
with ego. The ongoing journey of yoga is to take the restraints
which are mastered by a regular meditation practice (*sadhana*)
and transfer the peace and wisdoms engendered by that
practice to the circumstances of earthly life. We need to learn

even-heartedness and to operate as God's angels, no matter what circumstances are presented to us: it is all intended to strengthen us, to temper the metal of our single-edged, knife-edge path.

In this chapter, we are exploring calming even finer waves of restlessness, as the path becomes finer and finer to navigate, finding deeper and deeper stillness within as we progress. The aim is to find that inner stillness and to bring that stillness of peace into your actions, relationships and thoughts as you act in the external world. We must learn to embed and embody each experience of peace garnered in meditation in our daily lives. Rather than getting up after meditation and spilling all the gems received in that practice, we learn to carry that stillness with us as a living embodiment of peace. Thereby, meditation impacts directly on how we think, speak and act in the world and through striving to live a peaceful life.

An important text on the foundation of the path of Yoga *The Yogasutra,* was written by Patanjali around the second century CE. While the Bhagavad Gita and the Bible couch the truth in allegory, which can be ambiguously shrouded by successive translations as filtered through what was considered to be truth by the dominant thinking of each era, *The Yogasutra* describes the clear, exact method of the actual *how* to attain oneness with God. Patanjali enumerates a precise eight-step path to enlightenment, starting with how to behave as an aspiring yogi if you are seeking to realise the Self.

The first two steps detailed in *The Yogasutra* are the ten Dos and Don'ts (*yamas* and *niyamas*) of a moral code to operate in accordance with God's Law, (remarkably similar to Moses' Ten Commandments) which are the bedrock of living a spiritual life. The *yamas* are the how of acting in the external world: non-harming (*ahimsa*); truthfulness (*satya*); non-stealing (*asteya*); containment of vital life force, or as celibacy within a monastic setting (*brahmacharya*); and non-greed, non-possessiveness (*aparigraha*). The *niyamas* are the how of mastering one's inner world: purity of body and mind (*saucha*); contentment – mindfulness in the present moment and even-mindedness in all circumstances (*santosha*); self-discipline (*tapas*); personal introspection to weed out the ego's tendencies (*svadyaya*); devotion and surrender to God (*ishwara pranidhana*). The aspiring yogi must pull in the reins of the wild ego and learn to act as *if* he were enlightened. God loves a trier and is attracted to souls who try their best to act in accordance with His Laws, even if they falter many times, perseverance and sincerity are holy qualities.

Patanjali distilled yoga philosophy into one phrase: *chitta vritti nirodha*, which means the 'restraint (or neutralisation) of mental fluctuations'. *Chitta* is feeling but it also refers to the mental chatter of the mind (*manas*) which is never still unless we learn to nullify it through meditation. The smokescreen of emotional reactions and restless thoughts thrown by the ego consciousness is *chitta*. This is not to be confused with the pure feeling of the soul as happiness, joy and bliss for its own sake. Happiness is the natural feeling of the soul and requires no external result in order to feel happy. In contrast, the feeling of the ego is a restless broiling sea of emotion attached to selfish results – I am happy because I got the object of my desire or unhappy because my wishes were thwarted. The ego acts for personal gain and *chitta* is the excitable emotion of the heart as a direct result of fulfilment or disappointment in attaining selfish motives. *Chitta* refers to a continually restless storm of feeling and thoughts under the selfish, motive-led rule of the ego.

Nirodha means 'fluctuations or restless waves' and refers to the ego's attachment to the alternating peaks and troughs between happiness or unhappiness in response to events that arise in the drama of life.

Vritti means 'restraint, modification or neutralisation' and refers to the yogic practice of self-control in thought, word and deed. Mastering the practice of yoga techniques is the route by which we rein in the mind and restless emotion as listed by Patanjali: step 3 – mastering sitting still (*asana*) without bodily movement; step 4 – breath control (*pranayama*); step 5 – consciously withdrawing the life force from the physical body (*pratyahara*), pouring it into the vital torrent in the astral spine and upwards to awaken *ajna* and *sahasrara chakras*; step 6 – single-focused concentration (*dharana*) on God; step 7 – meditation proper (*dhyana*) where the body, mind and *chitta* have become still, absorbed in meditating on a manifestation of God as oneness, light, sound, peace, love, joy or stillness. Step 8 – total absorption in actual contact with God (*samadhi*) when the soul overcomes all restlessness and has attained such inner stillness and peace that God can be perceived within, without and everywhere. The final stage of *samadhi* has several stages of pure experience of God as separate (there is 'me' the perceiving soul, there is the perception and there is God) through to experiencing Oneness as God. Until a soul has attained the final stage through deep meditation, perseverance and yearning, the yogi will not be able to maintain holding onto the blissful experience of *samadhi*. The yogi may go in and out of *samadhi* for several years until this state can be maintained even as he or she acts in the world, with a dispassion and even-heartedness in all circumstances. Through even greater effort, dissolving all waves of ego restlessness and longer meditations, the soul will at last be able to achieve permanent union with God and true soul liberation from the bondage of incarnation (*kaivalya*).

In Chapter 1, we explored eliminating pairs of opposites of restless waves between ego result-driven desire for something in the external world as happiness or unhappiness with boredom as a flat-line between these two excitable experiences in order to win power from the ego in the battlefield of life away from the surface of the skin and the senses. Now, we are taking that focus deeper to neutralise the downward river of *prana* (life force) in the spine as it flows outward, into and becoming spent in all the many little streams and rivulets of engagement with the external world. Our vital force becomes 'watered down' and lost in the worldly attachments and the desires of the outwardly focused mind. Think of the external world like a desert mirage: it promises riches but in reality, it is a soul-sapping illusion which drains us of our vital current.

Sustained and empowered by the astral body, *prana* flows into the physical body through the back of the head. Individualised *prana* then becomes differentiated into five specific *prana* roles. *Prana* itself holds together the other four *pranas* to empower specific functions of the body: *apana* – excretes waste and toxins from the body and is a downward current; *vyana* – empowers the circulation of blood and encircles the whole body; *samana* – empowers digestion and the building of new cells, and is located in the midriff; and *udana* – controls the manufacture and dissolution of cells for specialised purposes in the body (such as skin, organ, hair, blood etc.).

When we arrived here from the Astral Realm to enliven our present physical body for habitation for this incarnation, our consciousness entered the crown of the head and descended the spine, down through each of the chakras until our consciousness was knotted into the body for a lifetime of experience. The physical body and family circumstances were a perfect match for all that you, as the indwelling soul, needed to learn in this lifetime (much as you may beg to differ, the cosmic attraction of the perfect parents and environment is exactly measured by karma as what you needed to learn). During the period of gestation and babyhood, our consciousness is in both the astral and physical worlds but increasingly we identify more with the cause and effect of the physical world as we become outwardly attached by sensory feedback. Thereby the true purpose in incarnating may be gradually forgotten as we become lost in *maya*. However, the strong thread of attraction of the soul to break free of karmically-induced incarnations still remains and that inner yearning calls us to turn away from the alluring baubles of sensory sensations and awake. This, then, is the battlefield with which the soul must engage in to return to permanent freedom in Spirit.

However, in the tug-of-war to reunite with the soul or to remain mesmerised by the Cosmic Delusion, the consciousness must overcome the two opposing currents in the spine: *prana* and *apana*. *Prana* is the ascending current in the astral spine which connects the soul with Spirit. *Apana* is the opposing descending current in the spine which draws the consciousness away from Spirit and out into matter. Therefore, as aspiring yogis, we must engage in battle every time we sit to meditate. The ego, using all manner of distractions, attempts to lure the awareness into the diverting currents of *apana*, to the surface of the skin and sensations of the external world. When the consciousness sides with the soul, we find our awareness uplifted in the current of *prana* in the spine, into increasingly expansive states of happiness, joy and peace.

The aim in engaging with this inner battle in the spine is to disengage with the senses and bodily sensation which are constantly sending a mind-boggling array of messages and stimulations. While the attention is in the sensory feedback, there can be no peace. The yoga breathing technique of Alternate Nostril Breath (*Nadi Shodanam*) (see Chapter 8) is an excellent method of neutralising the battle of the opposing currents *apana* (downward) and *prana* (upward) in the spine to bring stillness.

Alternate Nostril breath is a tranquillising practice which effectively balances the two opposing pathways of *ida* (left – moon energy) and *pingala* (right – sun energy), on either side of the spine. Then, as these become neutralised, the life force flows directly into the upward current in the spine. Through this technique, the consciousness can then win the battle for supremacy between *prana* and *apana*, and effectively 'calm' the battle. The consciousness can then ride the upward current of *prana* and reunite with Spirit once more.

Pranayama: Alternate Nostril Breath (*Nadi Shodhanam*) – Calming the Waves of Restlessness

Sit upright with the chin level. Lifting the right hand, place the thumb on the right nostril, ring finger and little finger on the left nostril. The other two fingers can be curled into the palm or placed on the brow (depending on your comfort). Grip lightly, without pinching, just below the bony bridge of the nose. Close the eyes.

Notice the sensation of the normal breath entering and exiting the nostrils. This can be felt as a vibration through the bridge of the nose. Is the vibration the same with the inhale and with the exhale?

Next time that you breathe out, close the right nostril with the thumb. Breathe in through the left nostril. Close the left nostril, and breathe out through the right.

Next breath: breathe in through the right nostril. Close the right nostril and breathe out through the left nostril.

Repeat this cycle of two breaths. Allow the inhale and exhale to be equal, long and smooth.

After a few breaths, introduce a pause after the inhale and, at the same time, holding the awareness on the brow. This pause is of indeterminate length as it is more important that you immerse your consciousness in the holding of the breath. In the pause, try to ride any waves of restlessness or distractions of the ego-mind.

Imagine that the breath is parting the Red Sea of restless thoughts to create a space between these two walls of water. The left and right balance in the centre at the brow.

As we go very deep in meditation, we learn to neutralise the two currents of *prana* and *apana* in the spine. The body then becomes very still. The rate of breathing and the heart rate

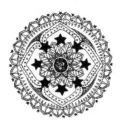

slow down. The physical body which tirelessly pumps red oxygenated blood around the body and removes toxins via the blood stream, finds that with the practice of neutralising the *apana-prana* currents, the heart beats very slowly and the breathing may stop for the space of a few breaths. This is the 'Breathless State' in which the body becomes very still. It is an indicator that the *apana-prana* currents are being neutralised as the normal restless processes of the body slow right down and for a period may stop altogether. As the pauses between the inhale and exhale, exhale and inhale naturally lengthen with the yoga breathing techniques, the body becomes sustained in those moments directly from *prana* (life force) and has no need to breathe. This is totally different from 'holding the breath' which takes conscious effort, feels very uncomfortable and can be dangerous for the body. In comparison, the breathless state is not sought, nor is the breath held consciously. The quiet of not-needing-to-breathe just arises with an accompanying calm. It is in the stillness of those breathless moments that you realise just how heavy, taxing and clunky the process of breathing is: like a set of bellows heaving air into and out of the body. It takes great effort, although we may not notice it, accustomed as we are to filtering this perception from our awareness. Nevertheless, the breath has been our constant reminder of being in bondage to a physical body, quite literally from birth.

During a tornado winds can be sucked by the whirling vortex to hundreds of miles per hour, but within the centre there is complete calm. Those that have survived a wide tornado sweeping directly over their shelter attest to the horrific wind followed by an utter stillness in the eye of the storm, and then deafening wind again as it passes away. In yogic terms, the eye of the storm is within the spine: external stimuli act as a great agitation on the senses and nerves of the physical, creating winds of restlessness in the mind and emotions. The dream-like physical world, and our sensory attachment to it, act as the storm of sensations, perceptions and emotions, which when we give it our attention, causes us to forget the peace that is within. When we start to draw our awareness back from the edges of the skin and from the sensory feedback, we win the first battle with the ego. Once our life force has successfully withdrawn to the spine, the second battle is epitomised by the *prana-apana* (ascending-descending) current in the spine itself for we are then battling for supremacy over the downward-outward facing ego consciousness. After ascending the current in the spine, the third battle is then highly localised within the *ajna* channel in the head, battling with very subtle ego traits.

In this chapter, we are focusing on that middle stage, the neutralisation of the ascending and descending currents in the spine. To withdraw the consciousness from the edges of the skin is a matter of choice: to stay outwardly immersed in the physical world or to go within. We can be in the surface of the skin, feeling what the body feels, or withdraw sensation further within the deep fascia which gives us proprioception feedback of where the body is in space. It is a matter of extricating consciousness from all that sensory feedback and to ignore all sensations. You learn to use willpower to 'unhook' the mind-attachment to sensory stimulation and decide to just feel what is in the spine: awareness of those upward and downward currents. *Prana* is felt as a coolness and *apana* is experienced as a warmth.

In the breathless state, you can experience great calm as if being in the eye of a storm: you experience a deep physical rest and calmness, with a heightened awareness that you are not the body. As I mentioned, in seeking to replicate a glorious experience in meditation this simply chases it out of our awareness. We just need to 'show up' and be present for each meditation. The Breathless State, though, is a wholesome way-marker that your practice is moving in the right direction.

The restless fluctuation stemming from our heart generator keeps us bound to a perception of separateness and an experience of duality. There may be occasions when the heart rate slows down or an imperceptible rhythm. This is usually accompanied by a 'weightiness' or sensation of dragging, which passes. The first time that my heart stopped entirely, I found myself in such surprising stillness and euphoria that I was totally taken aback. I had no idea just how much 'restlessness' the beating heart was causing in the body. It was as dramatically remarkable as if a pneumatic drill outside my window had just ceased. A wave of utter stillness and peace engulfed the smallness of my human body and lifted me into the vastness of expansive eternity brimming with peace. This timeless moment was soon eclipsed by the beating of the heart once more and the joyous peace-that-surpasses-understanding rolled back out of my awareness again. I have found that seeking these experiences pushes them further away. One just has to do the practice and be in each moment as it arises.

Even the breath and heartbeat are part of the restless and constant motion of this realm. The inhale and exhale and regularly beating heart operate automatically, without need for any conscious thought on our part. But still they bring a persistent vibration of motion which sets up a mild but persistent agitation within the bodily systems. Beneath these fluctuating waves of experience, there is a deep and still ocean of peace and soul calmness which expands into the infinite tranquillity of God.

The path of yoga is to become master of the body and mind. We learn to still the breath, to slow the beating heart and to withdraw awareness beyond the physical body to the more subtle states of being. This is achieved by using highly attuned awareness of the breath to pierce gross and subtle veils of restlessness (*koshas*) by withdrawing from external experience into internal expansiveness. It's only because we allow ourselves to become distracted by the allure and entertainments of the physical experience that we cannot be conscious that the perpetual peace already exists within.

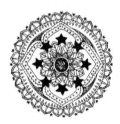

In order to find stillness, the body must be still. So fully engage with relaxing the body to set the foundation of the meditation on stillness. Seed tendencies of our karmic actions are stored in the brain and these are roasted or purified during this practice using alternate nostril breath and the *So Ham* mantra. The practice then goes on to offer the inhale into the exhale and the exhale into the inhale, so that selfishness, epitomised by the grasping of the breath, can be handed over. In life, we are used to grasping for this or that but we are learning here not to hold onto the breath, but immediately letting go of the sucking in of air in a greedy fashion as if air were a limited commodity.

Meditation on Stillness

Sit upright. Shift the weight from one buttock to the other so that you then sit still and become centred in the spine. Take a deep breath in, tense the body and hold the breath, exhale blowing away all bodily tension. Breathe in deeply, tense the body and hold, exhale blowing out all the cobwebs from the mind. Repeat once more.

Prayer: *Divine Mother, Jesus Christ and saints of all religions, teach me to extend thy love in my heart to all peoples; let me be helpful to all. Inspire me to love with your Divine Compassion for all beings. May I perceive the pulsing of Thy irrepressible life within all inanimate and animate matter. Om Shanti Peace.*

Be aware of the body breathing in and out. Watch the breathing of this body which is your vehicle for this incarnation.

You are not the body. Watch how it breathes.

You are not the breath either. You are simply observing.

Try to resist the urge to interfere with the breath: try to find something fresh and new in the breath on a process that you do thousands of times a day. Treat this as a mindfulness exercise to just observe. Perhaps your perspective is from the level of the brow or the back of the head. Is the breath smooth or ragged? Does the body expel all the breath in the lungs? Is the body breathing into the back body or the chest or the belly? Does the body want to have any natural pauses? Just observe this well-functioning body-machine doing what it wants to naturally do. Does the mind stay in the process or does it jump in and out? It doesn't matter how many times the mind disengages; it only matters how many times you bring it back.

Just watch whatever arises: perhaps it's the warmth of breath in the throat or the expansion of the alveoli in the lungs or a sense of calmness that arises as you watch the breath. Just be present to observe whatever arises.

Practise Alternate Nostril Breath for a few minutes.

Visualise that you are a mountain and continue with Alternate Nostril Breath: as you breathe in (through one nostril), air rushes up one slope. Hold the breath at the apex, and then exhale (through the opposite nostril) as air rushes down the other side of the mountain. Breathe in that ionised, cleansing air of the mountain and hold it at the summit. Breathe out a long exhale down the opposite slope. Perhaps the visualisation of breathing up and down the long mountain slope helps to slow the transit of the breath.

As you hold your breath at the summit, imagine that you are gazing out over the Himalayas or another mountainous range from a great height. Have a long calm inhale, a long pause at the brow (the summit) and a long slow exhale. Pull the focus of the eyes towards the brow on the pause and rein in the attention.

Release the hand posture (*mudra*) from the nose and let the hand relax. Continue to visualise the mountain with its strong base in the earth and your apex (head) in the heavens.

Visualise that channel of light in the spine with a firm base on the earth opening out on the brow chakra. Imagine that you are looking out over the high mountain tops in the Himalayas.

Observe that there is a subtle shift in the current in the spine with the inhale and with the exhale. There is also a physical shift in the hydraulics of the body with each breath (inhale creates pressure in the fluids of the body; exhale alleviates that pressure). Tune into that subtle movement of *prana-apana* in the spine. Just observe without trying to manipulate the breath.

Observe that as the body breathes in, there is an upward current in the spine. As the body breathes out, there is a downward current in the spine.

Continue to observe the breath as you introduce the *So Ham* mantra: mental mantra *So* with the inhale and mental mantra *Ham* with the exhale. Feel into a cool current that runs over the brain with the mental mantra *So*. A warm current flows over the brain with the mental mantra *Ham*.

You may think as you continue with *So Ham*: *I am not the body, I am He. I am not the ego, I am He.*

As a quiet develops you start to perceive the pure reflected light of the soul.

Imagine the still waters of consciousness. The *So* mantra blows over the surface waters of the mind and *Ham* resonates through the depths of the water. Although the surface can be calm, the depths may still have movement: let the mantra bring the surface and the depths to stillness.

Let the mantra recede.

Breathe in, offering the inhale as a gift into the exhale. Breathe out, offering the exhale into the forthcoming inhale. Even as the lungs are filling up, you are offering the prana (life force) into the exhale. Then as the body breathes out you are offering the out-breath into the forthcoming inhale. Let go of the sense of 'graspingness' in the breath. Just continue to offer the inhale into the exhale and the exhale into the inhale in this neutralisation practice.

Let go of the 'grasping' attachment to the body and the breath. Start to feel into something deeper. Pour the inhale into the exhale and exhale into the inhale. Perhaps your breath has become very shallow and slow. Perhaps you are starting to pour 'attachments', starting to feel empty.

Let go of the neutralising breath practice. Visualise a clear still pool of water. In the still water, you can see the clear reflected light of your own soul. You can see the pure crystalline reflection of your true self shining perfect and pure.

Feel into the depth of the water: feel the stillness. Feel into the depth of the earth, the stillness in the air. Feel into the stones of the quiet earth, only stillness. Feel into the stillness of the planet and the stars and the stillness of quiet expanded space.

I am the peace of the earth. I am the peace of stones. I am the peace of the stars. I am the peace of the outmost reaches of eternity. My peace spreads as stillness through all there is. My peace is the breath of saints. My peace is the breath of the stars. My stillness abounds and knows no end.

I am stillness. My peace expands from stillness. Like the birth of a new star, my heart opens and peace pours out. Feel the deep soul-rest that comes from stillness and overflowing peace.

Pour your peace onto the waters of the Earth. Pour your peace over your loved ones. Pour your peace over those who require your blessings. Visualise that they are bathed in peace.

Prayer: *Heavenly father, Divine mother, I stand before thee. Calm the storms of my restlessness. Bring thy stillness into this earthly life. May thy great peace descend and walk with me always. I give that peace to all. Om Shanti Peace.*

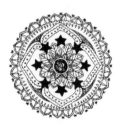

Reflect on this practice so that you carry this stillness, as the eye-of-the-storm, as you go about your normal everyday duties. They may be the same old tasks but *how* you do them will be different. Visualise being in the calm of the centre of the tornado as you act or visualise yourself with the surface of the pool, breathing softly, so that you can see yourself with the eyes of the soul. Or have your *So Ham* mantra playing mentally as you chop vegetables or walk the dog. Reflect on which practice you will take to move forward. Then you can take a practice, which is a seated meditation, and bring that focus and wisdom into how you act in daily life out in the world.

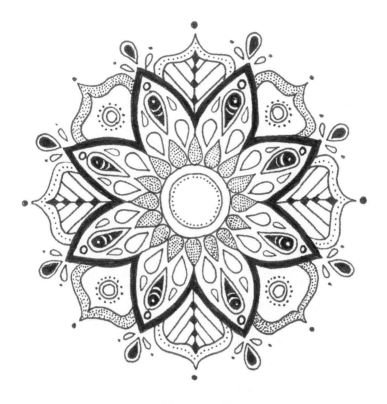

Chapter 15

The Cask of Silence

The kingdom of God is within you.
Luke 17:21

There is a deep silence within hitherto unplumbed and unknown to those at the mercy of the ego. We must meditate so deeply that we touch that inner silence. The peace arising from deep inner silence is the key signature that we have touched God. The Way is to still the waves of mental and emotional restlessness. In the thrall of the ego-consciousness, we would be perpetually tossed on the waves of life between the peaks of excitable happiness or miserable suffering or in the troughs of boredom between these waves. It is in boredom we can perceive that the ego thrives on drama, between escapism within the dream-existence as pleasure-seeking or wallowing in grief, anger or despondency. It was in my thirties, when I realised every three weeks or so, experiencing a boredom with nothing exciting going on, that I would manufacture some activity or drama in order to bring the excitement I craved, anything but boredom. I tell you this so that you too might recognise when you are manipulating a drama just for some gratification (all unwholesome truths bared here). The state of boredom is actually a window through which to see clearly the waves of restlessness, towering above, which threaten to engulf us if we don't play the ego game: *Get up, be sorrowful, be excited, be desirous of something in my make-believe world, be lost in my drama.* The ego craves excitement at all costs, it doesn't care if it drives us to be happy or sad, it only wants us to be blinkered and asleep in the *Divine Lila* (play).

Beneath all the waves of experience, there is deep peace. But if you live on the surface of life, in the grip of the ego-consciousness seeking its own selfish rewards and gains, you eventually come to realise that you are never quite at peace, wave-tossed between one drama and the next. In this chapter, we are diving deep into silence, the precursor to soul peace.

The deeper we dive into the soul in meditation, the deeper stillness is felt. But first we must still the body by eliminating all tension and restlessness from the muscles (see Chapter 3). Full deep breathing, inhaling and tensing, and exhaling and relaxing the body a few times, expels restless 'static' from the body until the muscles relax (except as required for upright stability). After you have succeeded in purging restlessness from the body, forget the body. Turn your attention to Watching the Breath (see Chapter 1) and guard against each twitch or any slight tensing of the body. There is a fine line between moving outwards into body consciousness to let go of any perceived tension, while at the same time observing release of any tension that may have crept in, at a mental distance from the body. Dropping body consciousness takes practice. When you can let go of attachment to the sensations of the body and go within, dive deep and expand the consciousness. This may seem like a conundrum: to go within at the same time as expansion, but the withdrawal from body consciousness is an awareness shift into super-conscious expanded space, beyond the domain of the earthly conscious mind. When you can dive deeper yet and feel your consciousness in every pore of the universe, in every flower, every heart, every star, then you are entering Cosmic Consciousness.

The second mastery in meditation is from being at the mercy of restless thoughts. Dive so deeply in meditation that you can ignore all the wiles of the ego, presented as alluring distractions. It takes practice to carve out a sacred space within the mind and push back the edges where restless thought threads cannot enter. In physical yoga, a *drishti* (focal point for the eyes) is employed in order to sustain a balance pose: if the eyes are fixed on one point, balance is steady, if the eyes flick around, balance is poor. Likewise, in meditation, we learn to keep the mental gaze focused on and slowly expand the mind space, ignoring anything else at the edges of your awareness. You may like to imagine that you are blowing a huge soap bubble: a slow steady exhale into the soap ring inflates a rainbow-bright bubble around you, pushing back the air. Or imagine that you are pushing back the Red Sea of thoughts. Create a mental haven of stillness within the mind and then dive deeper.

When restless thoughts have been banished to the edges, a silence is found. Then you realise how noisy the mental static was: it makes you wonder how you could think clearly at all. Diving deeper, silence is transformed into pure intuitive feeling and our heart becomes an inner haven of peace where we may find God. Peace is a deeper quality than silence and is the first inner manifestation of God in meditation. As we advance still deeper in meditation, peace expands into a deeper experience of bliss. Bliss is a deeper manifestation of God than peace and indicates that we are experiencing *Samadhi* (highest state of meditation). However, we must persistently dive deeper in meditation until the bliss of Samadhi does not slip away as we act in the divine drama for then we can become unruffled consciousness in the midst of all circumstances that life presents. Such is the challenge of an earthly incarnation.

So we learn to still the body, have that silent breath, still the thoughts so that all restlessness is stilled and then there is deep quiet within. You may like to visualise the Sea of Restlessness as being tossed on the wave of one experience or another, if you emotionally attach to it. Instead, you can see the waves as just the divine play and 'step back' from being caught up in it all. Meditation gives us that distance, that objectivity to dive into silence. All the wonders of the universe are heard in that silence. The strains of human hearing can hear nine octaves and there are physical sounds above and below that the physical ears cannot register. But beyond that there are the musical sounds of the chakras which make a beautiful symphony in themself: in the base chakra (*muladhara*), there is a humming sound of the bee; in the sacral chakra (*svadisthana*), there is a sound like a flute; *manipura* (navel) has a sound like a harp or violin; *anahata* (heart) sounds like a gong or a bell; the throat chakra (*vishuddhi*) sounds like running water; and at the back of the head (*ajna chakra*) an orchestra of all astral sounds can be heard as the deep humming of the cosmic engine or OM. (When I first heard rushing water in meditation, I thought a tap was running so I had to get up and ascertain where it was coming from, but no tap was on. The same thing happened three times in a row before I was convinced that it was an astral sound and not a physical one. That's how convincingly like the sound of rushing water it is, not simply imagination.) As you advance in meditation, one or all of the chakras of the astral body become clear and you may witness astral music as it opens. However, it takes deep practice to still the body, mind and feeling to such a point that you can hear astral sound.

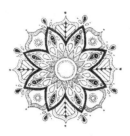

Meditation: *Shanti* (Peace) Mantra

Come into your meditation posture by sitting upright. Visualise the spine as a hollow shaft of rainbow light.

Connect to that channel of Divine Light that is always flowing in through the crown of the head.

Prayer: *Divine Spirit, make me receptive to Thy peace, let me feel Thy peace in every fibre of my being, fill my heart to overflowing with Thy peace. Om Shanti Peace.*

Be aware of that shaft of light in the spine. Allow the skylight of your crown to open to let in spiritual sunlight, flooding the hollow shaft in the spine with Divine Light.

Breathe in that flood of pure white light through the crown of the head in a long peaceful breath. Breathe out a calming balm of peacefulness in a long breath over the body.

Use the mental mantra *OM* on the inhale and *shanti* (meaning Peace) on the exhale. *OM* calms the nerves of the body and *shanti* is soothing balm over the body.

The mental mantra *OM* with the inhale, brings a cooling peacefulness over the brain. *Shanti* brings a coolness within the skull with the exhale, as a wave of light flowing through the brain.

Incorporate a pause after the inhale. Receive a flood of light through the crown with OM on the inhale. Feel a sense of gratitude as you hold the breath. Then the long smooth exhale with *shanti*.

Shift your practice to visualise the shaft of light into the astral spine containing the rainbow light of the six main chakras and the spine flooded with light from the crown chakra, *sahasrara*, as the light of a thousand suns. Mental mantra OM on the inhale, stimulating the chakras and *shanti* on the exhale stimulating that flow of the spiritual light of a thousand suns through the crown of the head. Feel as though your crown has opened up to become a larger space.

Visualise the mental mantra *shanti* vibrating through the heart as calming wind. OM on the inhale shatters any chain of self-created limitation. Mental mantra *shanti* brings a balm of peace throughout the heart.

Visualise a still pool of water in a forest, reflecting the stillness of the forest. There is a perfect mirror reflection of the forest and the sky in the still pool. There is a slight rippling of the surface of the water as you breathe in and out. Learn to breathe in and out with a smooth breath so that the surface of the pool remains unrippled, as smooth as a mirror reflecting the trees and the open sky.

The surface of the pool becomes a sheet of light. The inhale and exhale are long and smooth, with pauses between the breaths. Learn to hold onto that expression of peace in the pauses after the inhale and after the exhale so that surface of the pool remains as a still sheet of light.

Learn to contain that fullness of peace. Learn to ride the awareness of any restlessness that tries to intrude. You are holding it back, as if holding back the wall of water in the Red Sea. Allow your focus not to be on any restlessness if it arises, but merely the containment of a growing Peacefulness.

Breathe in, the water remains as a sheet of light, containing the peacefulness. Breathe out, allowing the peacefulness to flow out over your entire being.

Let the surface of the water be an indicator of attaining the vibration of peace. You are in the University of Life. You are in training, and each breath is a fresh do-over to manufacture peacefulness and to hold onto it. Each breath is a fresh attempt to tune into the vibration of peace that is always present, flowing through you, and to hold onto it.

Congratulate yourself for each second that you hold the peace vibration. Each breath is a fresh attempt as you gain your spiritual muscles by trying.

Open your spiritual eyes to look at the pool of light in front of you. Notice the forest around you as stillness. You are the epicentre of that stillness.

That peacefulness and stillness constantly flows through all of creation and through you, realise that the flow of peace flows in to your heart. Allow the forest scene to recede and become aware of being expansive in space.

In all directions, there is only peace emanating from within.

Use the mental mantra *Om Shanti* to expand your consciousness, spreading over the whole of space.

Become open to receive that frequency of God's peace that is constantly flowing in. You are buoyed up and supported by that flow of peace. If you receive with a tiny thimble, that will be filled. If you receive with a cup, that will be filled. If you receive with the whole of your being, you will be filled, filled with the peace of God.

Allow the inner recesses of your heart to open to that peace flowing through your being. As if you were a flower receiving the blessing of rays of spiritual light. Drink in that spiritual light and peace.

That vision of yourself as a flower is superimposed upon your physical frame. Breathing in peace and breathing out peace. Visualise your peace flowing around the world, bringing solace and comfort into receptive hearts.

Breathe in peace and breathe peace out, upon the waters of

the world.

Bring praying hands to the heart and finish by chanting *Om Shanti, Shanti, Shanti.*

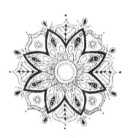

All the wonders of creation are heard in silence.

Being silent is conducive to our spiritual unfoldment. With so much busyness in our daily life, how can we develop more silence? Gandhi took one day a week as a day of silence: this was more than just non-speaking, he used the time to be quiet within, in seclusion from his pressing engagements. Those who became spiritual masters won this by spending a great deal of time in silence or being silent within. Those who step into a practice of silence find it so nurturing that they wouldn't want to go back to clamour. It is restorative to have a day a week to go within to find peace, a day between you and God. Perhaps, you may think about having more periods of silence in your life. Silence is the price of wisdom.

Silence begets more silence. Are there times in your life when potential moments of silence are filled with useless noise? Are there disturbances such as TV, radio, podcasts, listening to music, social media, chatting on the phone or video chat, which you could reduce or banish one day a week? It may be wise to inform your household in advance that you are having a morning or a day of silence. I would invite you to give it a go – silence is a really fulfilling practice in itself.

What constitutes silence in your daily life? Silence is more than just non-speaking. It is practising inner quiet: letting go of agitated thoughts and emotions, and foregoing useless distractions for quiet reflection or meditation. Free up as much time as you can to have silence inside and out. Perhaps you can aim to contain the inner quiet touched in meditation for as long as you can sustain afterwards. It is worth noting that speech spills those pearls of wisdom and pierces the silence which is garnered in meditation. An Indian saying illustrates this well: it is as if you have milked the cow but then jumped up and kicked over the bucket. In meditation, we 'empty' ourselves of worldly attachments and fill with life force (*prana*), calm, divine peace and wisdom: the 'milk' of meditation. The process of meditating isn't just something that you do, walk away from and return to fractiously acting in the world. Aspire to hold the pearls that you attain in meditation going for as long as possible when you act once more in the world. You may like to timetable reminders to touch back into calm or silence or peace at some point throughout the day – perhaps set a Tibetan bell app to chime at regular intervals or stick post-its at strategic points in the home or office. I know someone who writes an OM symbol on the palm of his hand to remind him to have little mini-meditations – his productivity actually improved by factoring in mindfulness moments at work.

Early in our meditation practice, it is all bells and whistles – tangible encouragement that you are on the right track. As you go deeper these experiences occur less frequently. This isn't because your practice is ineffectual but to teach you to persevere, not to give up in the face of another aspect of the ego that is seeking an obvious result. Your practice will still be peppered with sudden illuminations, of stillness, of the presence of God as light, great love or deep peace, which arise just when you expect it least. This is to teach you to meditate and follow the practice steadfastly just because it is right, because it makes you feel calm or peaceful or well or happy. We should not seek these bolts from the blue (as that is the ego creeping in looking for results) but divine blessings are given to us, just when we are not looking for it. These pearls of wisdom that you receive in inner silence are divine gifts, something to be kept private between you and God. If we speak about these experiences before we have had time to assimilate and embed then in our consciousness, these are spilled and spoiled. Hold these gems precious within your heart of hearts. These wisdoms grow within us a divine garden of inner riches, far more beautiful that any impermanent bauble of this world: but only if we allow them to take root and become established as who we are. These precious moments will sustain you in the inevitable barren periods in your practice when things go a bit dry or mechanical, when nothing seems to be happening. If you are ever assailed by inner doubts, know that this is just an aspect of ego-consciousness. These are the times to revisit your inner treasure trove of divine blessings. These gifts will encourage you to keep going in your meditation practice until it is once more uplifting each time that you sit.

We all go through periods when we appear to be plodding through a dark tunnel feeling very alone which can persist for weeks sometimes. Just know that you are shifting a load of karma, which presents as moods, heaviness on the soul and lightless, apparently rudderless meditations. In these difficult times we should seek the refuge of meditation and dive deeper. Use the *sadhana* practice to lift you out of whatever is burning off your soul and pour your heart out to God and with all the love of your soul, ask for help. Hand over the burden to the holy 'feet' of the Divine. Keep praying with all your soul and you will be answered (this can take fifteen minutes of heartfelt prayer or much longer but don't give up for you will feel lighter afterwards). I invite you to lay all your weight at the feet of our Father/Mother who loves us dearly. At some point in eternity, God dreamed you into existence and that makes you special, loved beyond measure. Speak to He who is your Heavenly Father or She who is the Divine Mother, with all your heart and soul for that is the Way. Bleeding feet, open heart, we all climb the final summit to stand clear, upright and smiling, bathed in the glory of Divine Love.

How will we know when we have touched God? When I was seven years old, the teacher opened a discussion about what God looked like. All the other kids were expounding the popular belief of God as a remote, stern fatherly figure on a throne with a long biblical beard. I sat silently holding my vision of God. The teacher then asked us to draw God. It took me all of two minutes to draw vast emanating golden light throughout all of the cosmos with a yellow crayon, the nearest colour I had to what I could see internally. First finished, I took it to the teacher. 'What's that?' she asked. 'God,' I said. 'No, it's not,' she replied. 'Yes it is,' I instantly said, 'God isn't a person, God is Light.' The poor woman sat open mouthed. I laugh when I look back at that moment. But what does God look like? Or how will we know God? Blossoming inner peace is one of the key signatures of God but others are Light, Love, Sound, Wisdom, Grace and Bliss. This is not a one-sided relationship with the Divine. Meditation is where we learn to listen and become attuned to the vibration of God. Prayer is where we speak to God.

To find the kingdom of the Peace-God, we must look within. We must cast out all restlessness of body, mind and spirit in order to draw near to that kingdom. It is our restlessness of consciousness which sets us apart. In this meditation, we use a technique to eliminate restlessness and seek the inner cask of silence.

Meditation on Silence

Breathe in deeply, tense the whole body, hold (gazing towards the brow chakra), then breathe out with a sigh, letting go of tension and 'static' from the body. Repeat once more. Repeat a third time, using the out-breath to let go of restlessness of mind and feeling.

Prayer: *Divine Father, Divine Mother, Jesus Christ, Paramahansa Yogananda, St Francis, saints of all religions, I stand before thee. Bless me with Thy deepest awareness of Peace. Bless me that Thy peace may flow, stilling all the waves of restlessness. Let me become as a little child, joyous and without guile. Let me experience Thy deepest peace, fill me with Thy peace that surpasses understanding. Om Shanti Peace.*

Watch the Breath, while at the same time practising the *So Ham* mental mantra. Remind yourself that you are neither the body, nor the clunking mechanical breath. If you find the ego has jumped in, anticipating the next inhale or exhale, step back again to observe. By degrees eliminate ego-consciousness.

Allow any pauses to develop in the breath. The deeper your attention, the more spaces arise between inhale-exhale or exhale-inhale.

Just observe. The process is waiting until the soul consciousness takes over and the ego consciousness steps back.

Mental mantra *So Ham* rides on the breath. The breath is beneath the mantra. The body is beneath the breath.

Mentally affirm: *When I was a child, I did childish things; now I lay aside those childish attachments and seek who I AM.*

Sink deeper in meditation. Let go of the *So Ham* mantra. Drop deep into quiet.

Take your consciousness in listening deeply to the space between the ears or out into expanded space. Without expectation. Just listen.

Tune out the 'white noise' of the ears (that is just the singing of the electrical nerves of the physical body). Listen deeply to the rhythms of the body until they recede. Go behind those sounds.

Open the throat slightly. Let the gentle drops of ambrosia drip into your receptive heart. Visualise the heart petals rotating to face upward towards spiritual sunlight, the petals eagerly drinking the elixir of peace.

Come back to listening deeply.

Notice where you are listening from: the back of the head, the neck, the head or the heart.

Go deeper into inner silence. As the petals of the heart opens, silence pours out: silence of the heavens, silence of the stars, silence of the further most reaches of space, the silence of inner beauty, perhaps bringing with it a fragrance of peace. A deep inner peace is behind that silence.

Drink in the silence. Become like a flower after a drought, eagerly soaking up the rain.

Drink deeply of your inner cask of silence. Let go of any impediments to experiencing that silence (any tightness or attachment within and realising, let it go).

Let go of childish things: imagine holding them as bright balloons, floating away as you let go of the strings.

Affirmation: *I let go of all restlessness and the trials of life for, I rule in my refuge of inner silence.*

Let the affirmation float your consciousness into deeper silence and into peace, as tangible direct contact with the Divine.

Let go of the affirmation and allow each moment to bring a fresh flow of peace.

Speak in your inner heart to the Divine as your dearest friend.

Into the silence, come back into your earthly existence for you have a job to do, not any of the earthly duties but simply to act in the world from this place of peace. Blessed are the peacemakers. We are manufacturing peace and bring that peace out into our daily activities.

Send peace to your loved ones, bathing them in the peace emanating from your soul.

Send peace to your neighbours, your town, your nation and all the nations of the world.

Send peace to all: from the humblest ant to the vast blue whale and to all humankind. Send special blessings of peace to the peace-makers of the planet seeking to bring harmony between peoples, for together we herald the harmony of the Golden Age of Earth. Bathe the whole planet in peace.

Prayer: *Divine Father, Jesus Christ, Paramahansa Yogananda, St Francis and saints of all religions, we bow to thee. Awaken us that we may know Thy Peace, that peace that flows from the cask of silence found in deep meditation. Bathe us in Thy Peace, Thy wisdom, Thy harmony now and always, Om Shanti Peace Amen.*

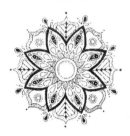

Try to contain this peace as you go about your activities. Mentally recite the *So Ham* Mantra as you do your humble earthly deeds or if you lose that, swing back into it frequently throughout the day. Alternatively, use the affirmation:

I let go of all restlessness and the trials of life, for I rule in the refuge of my inner silence.

Developing Peace Within

A Message from the Author

Peace awaits those who have the courage to dive within and seek it. That first touch of peace is sure to prove so nourishing that you are certain to yearn for its solace, longing with such a passion and dedication that you do find lasting inner peace. So keep diving within! Don't be put off by those petty little desires for trinkets that the pseudo-self dangles before us. We all know how hollow, entangling and empty it will be to actually own those earthly baubles and toys: the only ego satisfaction is in whipping our consciousness to seek that which is impermanent and unsatisfying, and then it's off again on the perpetual hunt for something else.

Having tasted peace as a divine elixir, divine fragrance, inner stillness, a boundless sphere, peace rays or whichever 'route' yielded peace for you, persevere with that. I invite you to dive deeper into that avenue to peace which most appealed to you, using the meditation techniques to amplify an actual experience of peace.

Peace arrives as a calmness, then within that calmness, it further develops into peace. Even deeper than peace, we find an expansive, eternal joy in meditation. Peace is a sure sign of communing with the Great Oneness. Once the ego has become quiet, *the peace of God which passeth all understanding* (Philippians 4:7) arises within. Then, we truly know without a shadow of a doubt that we are soul, and as a soul-spark of that Great Oneness, we *are* God. All dual awareness of 'me, mine, I' dissolves into universal oneness, spread through eternity as peace, light, love and joy.

Whether you persevere until you reach the ultimate liberation of the soul in oneness with the peace of God (*kaivalya*) or are simply seeking to bring rest and calm between the warring factions of the restless ego consciousness, I urge you to keep on keeping on in daily meditation and you will receive what you have spiritually yearned for. Listen to that incessant inner yearning and spiritual determination (*svadharma*) for that is the voice of the soul and it will lead you to more quiet, increasing calmness beyond the deepest balm of peace imaginable. Once you come to the realisation that nothing really stands in the way to peace, all remnants of ego-restlessness will be nothing but a shadowy dream, when upon waking in the sunshine of spirit, we can see that that which seemed so firm and immoveable, is revealed as an insubstantial dream, with no more hold over us than a wisp of cloud.

My richest blessings go with you as you soldier on in the battlefield of everyday life to manifest peace in the ordinary interactions with family and friends and mundane activities of Earth, rallying your soul forces against the ever-diminishing bluster of the ego.

If you would like to connect with other books that I have coming in the near future, please visit my website for news on upcoming works, yoga blog posts, articles, podcasts, courses, retreats and events, and sign up for my newsletter: https://www.living-lightly.co.uk. You can listen to my voice guiding you through some of the meditations in this book from my website. Also, if you have a few moments, I would welcome your review of this book on your favourite online site for feedback.

May you find peace in your mind, peace in your heart and peace in your soul.

Warmest love,

Om Shanti Peace.

Jenny Light

Acknowledgements

I am deeply grateful to my friends and daughters for their help with this book. I thank Neil Campbell and my daughter Ashley Brown, for their comments and invaluable support in proofing this book. For the beautiful artwork, I thank my daughter Lesley Brown, for meditating on the subject of each chapter, designing and illustrating a beautiful peace mandala for each one. I also thank graphic artist and friend, Suze McCallum, for her evocative cover design.

I am grateful for the kind permission to reprint from *'Where There is Light'* and *'Metaphysical Meditations'* by Paramahansa Yogananda by Self-Realization Fellowship, Los Angeles, U.S.A.. To my guru, Paramahansa Yogananda, my deepest gratitude for his untold blessings. Without the faithful support and guidance from my guru, this book could not have been written. I am merely the vehicle by which his words pour through.

Finally, I am grateful to you, dear reader, for a book without a reader is a dry and lifeless thing. I pray that you receive the richest of blessings, that you become illumined with peace, within, without and that you walk the path of calmness perpetually carrying that torch of eternal peace to touch the lives of those whom you meet. Alight with inner peace, with you in your small corner and I in mine, we change the world, one heart at a time.

Together, let us shine that peace to all.

About the Author

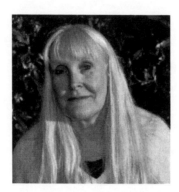

Jenny Light is a Scottish Yogi born in 1963 who had a kundalini awakening as a small child. *Awakening the Lotus of Peace* draws on her personal experiences and those of her students as a stage by stage guide to overcoming ego delusions to find the true self within. Jenny has over twenty years' experience teaching yoga, is a 1000-hour member of the Independent Yoga Network, a disciple of Paramahansa Yogananda and has been immersed in yoga as a way of life for fifty years. She has an MA in Psychology and Philosophy and spent twenty-five years in education as an Additional Support Needs teacher. She is a blogger, author, podcaster and writer for many yoga and Mind Body Spirit magazines.

In her previous books, Jenny expounded yoga philosophy and yoga meditations on the twenty-six qualities of the soul in *Divine Meditations: Twenty-six Qualities of the Bhagavad Gita* (Mantra Books 2019) and charted her autobiographical journey from extreme sensitivity in her self-help book *Living Lightly: A Journey through Chronic Fatigue Syndrome (M.E.)* (Ayni Book 2016).

Jenny lives in Ayrshire with her husband, enjoying time with her five grandchildren and painting seascapes.

Previous Books by Jenny Light

Divine Meditations: 26 Spiritual Qualities of the Bhagavad Gita by
Jenny Light
Mantra Books 2019
Discover your Divine heritage through meditation. *Divine Meditations: 26 Spiritual Qualities of the Bhagavad Gita* is an inspirational, spiritual workbook which unravels the veils covering the light of the Self, by focusing on the 26 God-like qualities, such as purity, compassion and ahimsa (non-harming), using intuitional wisdom, pranayama, mantra, meditations and prayers. Structured in four parts and focusing upon meditation in reference to Patanjali's eightfold path, the Bhagavad Gita and the spiritual aspirant, the 26 qualities and how to assume them and transcending the Cosmic Illusion through Yoga breathing (*pranayama*) to focus prana (life force); Meditating to achieve a super-conscious state to find lasting happiness within.

This is a fine book, so good it should anchor the spiritual wing of your personal library.
Jack Hawley, author of *The Bhagavad Gita: a Walkthrough for Westerners*.

I recommend this book by Jenny Light to all those who are seeking spiritual Truth.
Stephen Sturgess, author of *The Yoga Book* and *The book of Chakras and Subtle Bodies*.

Living Lightly: A Journey through Chronic Fatigue Syndrome
(M.E.) by Jenny Light
Ayni Books 2016

An autobiographical, self-help guide for those with Chronic Fatigue Syndrome (M.E.). This is a light-hearted reflection on the lessons learnt from the condition and teaches clear techniques on self-healing, breathing, meditation, positive thinking, affirmation, supplements and raw-food diet to recover full health.

Jenny Light has got a 'light' on the problem of Chronic Fatigue Syndrome... she takes you on an inward journey to full health, through healthy living, exercises and therapies that can be used to overcome Chronic Fatigue Syndrome.

Jan De Vries, nature-cure doctor and author of *By Appointment Only* series.

Inspirational Reading

Paramahansa Yogananda, *God Talks with Arjuna: The Bhagavad Gita*, 1955, Self Realization Fellowship.

Paramahansa Yogananda, *Metaphysical Meditations*, 2012, Self Realization Fellowship.

Paramahansa Yogananda, *Where There Is Light*, 2015, Self Realization Fellowship.

Richard Hittleman, *Yoga Twenty-eight Day Exercise Plan* 1969, Workman Publishing Company, New York.

Swami Sivananda, *The Bhagavad Gita*. World Wide Web (WWW) Edition: 2000, The Divine Life Society.

Swami Niranjanananda Saraswati, *Prana and Pranayama*, Bihar School of Yoga, Bihar, India 2009

Swami Sri Yukteswar Giri, *The Holy Science*, 1949, Self Realization Fellowship.

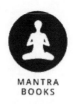

MANTRA
BOOKS

EASTERN RELIGION & PHILOSOPHY

We publish books on Eastern religions and philosophies. Books
that aim to inform and explore the various traditions that began in
the East and have migrated West.
If you have enjoyed this book, why not tell other readers by
posting a review on your preferred book site.

Recent bestsellers from MANTRA BOOKS are:

The Way Things Are
A Living Approach to Buddhism
Lama Ole Nydahl
An introduction to the teachings of the Buddha, and how to make
use of these teachings in everyday life.
Paperback: 978-1-84694-042-2 ebook: 978-1-78099-845-9

Back to the Truth
5000 Years of Advaita
Dennis Waite
A demystifying guide to Advaita for both those new to, and those
familiar with this ancient, non-dualist philosophy from India.
Paperback: 978-1-90504-761-1 ebook: 978-184694-624-0

Shinto: A celebration of Life
Aidan Rankin
Introducing a gentle but powerful spiritual pathway reconnecting
humanity with Great Nature and affirming all aspects of life.
Paperback: 978-1-84694-438-3 ebook: 978-1-84694-738-4

In the Light of Meditation
Mike George
A comprehensive introduction to the practice of meditation and the spiritual principles behind it. A 10 lesson meditation programme with CD and internet support.
Paperback: 978-1-90381-661-5

A Path of Joy
Popping into Freedom
Paramananda Ishaya
A simple and joyful path to spiritual enlightenment.
Paperback: 978-1-78279-323-6 ebook: 978-1-78279-322-9

The Less Dust the More Trust
Participating in The Shamatha Project, Meditation and Science
Adeline van Waning, MD PhD
The inside-story of a woman participating in frontline meditation research, exploring the interfaces of mind-practice, science and psychology.
Paperback: 978-1-78099-948-7 ebook: 978-1-78279-657-2

I Know How To Live, I Know How To Die
The Teachings of Dadi Janki: A warm, radical, and life-affirming view of who we are, where we come from, and what time is calling us to do
Neville Hodgkinson
Life and death are explored in the context of frontier science and deep soul awareness.
Paperback: 978-1-78535-013-9 ebook: 978-1-78535-014-6

Living Jainism

An Ethical Science
Aidan Rankin, Kanti V. Mardia
A radical new perspective on science rooted in intuitive awareness
and deductive reasoning.
Paperback: 978-1-78099-912-8 ebook: 978-1-78099-911-1

Ordinary Women, Extraordinary Wisdom

The Feminine Face of Awakening
Rita Marie Robinson
A collection of intimate conversations with female spiritual
teachers who live like ordinary women, but are engaged with their
true natures.
Paperback: 978-1-84694-068-2 ebook: 978-1-78099-908-1

The Way of Nothing

Nothing in the Way
Paramananda Ishaya
A fresh and light-hearted exploration of the amazing reality of
nothingness.
Paperback: 978-1-78279-307-6 ebook: 978-1-78099-840-4

Readers of ebooks can buy or view any of these bestsellers by
clicking on the live link in the title. Most titles are published in
paperback and as an ebook. Paperbacks are available in traditional
bookshops. Both print and ebook formats are available online.

Find more titles and sign up to our readers' newsletter at
http://www.johnhuntpublishing.com/mind-body-spirit.
Follow us on Facebook at https://www.facebook.com/OBooks
and Twitter at https://twitter.com/obooks.